BLACKWELL

UNDERGROUND CLINICAL VIGNETTES

OBSTETRICS AND GYNECOLOGY, 3E

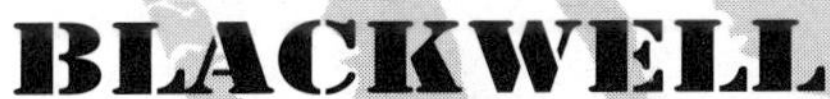

BLACKWELL

UNDERGROUND CLINICAL VIGNETTES

OBSTETRICS AND GYNECOLOGY, 3E

VIKAS BHUSHAN, MD
Series Editor
University of California, San Francisco, Class of 1991
Diagnostic Radiologist

VISHAL PALL, MD, MPH
Series Editor
Internist and Preventive Medicine Specialist
Government Medical College, Chandigarh – Panjab University – India, Class of 1997
Graduate School of Biomedical Sciences at UTMB Galveston, MPH, Class of 2004

TAO LE, MD
University of California, San Francisco, Class of 1996

KYONG UN CHONG
Joan C. Edwards School of Medicine, West Virginia, Class of 2005

SHARATCHANDRA BIDARI, MBBS, MD
Shri B.M. Patil Medical College, Bijapur, India, Class of 1996
Diagnostic Radiologist

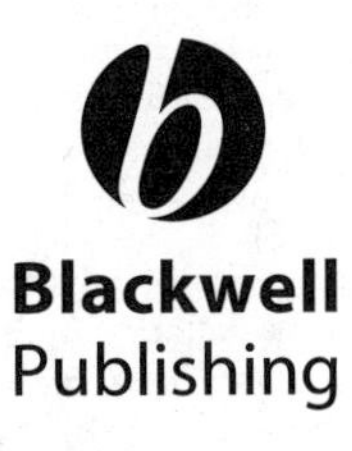

Blackwell Publishing, Inc., 350 Main Street, Malden, Massachusetts 02148-5018, USA
Blackwell Publishing Ltd, 9600 Garsington Road, Oxford OX4 2DQ, UK
Blackwell Publishing Asia Pty Ltd, 550 Swanston Street, Carlton, Victoria 3053, Australia

05 06 07 08 5 4 3 2 1

ISBN-13: 978-1-4051-0423-4
ISBN-10: 1-4051-0423-6

Library of Congress Cataloging-in-Publication Data

Obstetrics and gynecology / Vikas Bhushan . . . [et al.]. — 3rd ed.
p. ; cm. — (Blackwell underground clinical vignettes)
Rev. ed. of: OB/GYN / author, Vikas Bhushan. 2nd ed. 2002.
"USMLE step 2 review."
ISBN-13: 978-1-4051-0423-4 (pbk. : alk. paper)
ISBN-10: 1-4051-0423-6 (pbk. : alk. paper)
1. Gynecology—Case studies. 2. Obstetrics—Case studies. 3. Physicians—Licenses—United States—Examinations—Study guides. I. Bhushan, Vikas. II. Bhushan, Vikas. OB/GYN. III. Series: Blackwell's underground clinical vignettes.
[DNLM: 1. Genital Diseases, Female—Case Reports. 2. Genital Diseases, Female—Problems and Exercises. 3. Pregnancy Complications—Case Reports. 4. Pregnancy Complications—Problems and Exercises. WP 18.2 O137 2005]

RG106.B48 2005
618′.076—dc22

2005007939

A catalogue record for this title is available from the British Library

Acquisitions: Nancy Anastasi Duffy
Development and Production: Debra Murphy
Cover and Interior Design: Leslie Haimes
Typesetter: Graphicraft in Quarry Bay, Hong Kong
Printed and bound by Capital City Press in Berlin, VT

For further information on Blackwell Publishing, visit our website:
www.blackwellmedstudent.com

NOTICE

The indications and dosages of all drugs in this book have been recommended in the medical literature and conform to the practices of the general community. The medications described do not necessarily have specific approval by the Food and Drug Administration for use in the diseases and dosages for which they are recommended. The package insert for each drug should be consulted for use and dosage as approved by the FDA. Because standards for usage change, it is advisable to keep abreast of revised recommendations, particularly those concerning new drugs.

The authors of this volume have taken care that the information contained herein is accurate and compatible with the standards generally accepted at the time of publication. Nevertheless, it is difficult to ensure that all the information given is entirely accurate for all circumstances. The publisher and authors do not guarantee the contents of this book and disclaim any liability, loss, or damage incurred as a consequence, directly or indirectly, of the use and application of any of the contents of this volume.

The publisher's policy is to use permanent paper from mills that operate a sustainable forestry policy, and which has been manufactured from pulp processed using acid-free and elementary chlorine-free practices. Furthermore, the publisher ensures that the text paper and cover board used have met acceptable environmental accreditation standards.

CONTENTS

CONTRIBUTORS

Alireza Khazaeizadeh, MD
Shiraz University School of Medicine, Class of 1995
Associate Professor, Department of Biochemistry, St. Luke's University School of Medicine

Hoang Nguyen, MD, MBA
Northwestern University, Class of 2001

Faculty Reviewer

Véronique Taché, MD
UCLA School of Medicine/ Class of 2003
UC Davis Medical Center, Department of Obstetrics and Gynecology

ACKNOWLEDGMENTS

Throughout the production of this book, we have had the support of many friends and colleagues. Special thanks to our support team including Andrea Fellows, Anastasia Anderson, Srishti Gupta, Anu Gupta, Mona Pall, Jonathan Kirsch, and Chirag Amin. For prior contributions we thank Gianni Le Nguyen, Tarun Mathur, Alex Grimm, Sonia Santos, and Elizabeth Sanders.

For submitting comments, corrections, editing, proofreading, and assistance across all of the vignette titles in all editions, we collectively thank:

Tara Adamovich, Carolyn Alexander, Kris Alden, Henry E. Aryan, Lynman Bacolor, Natalie Barteneva, Dean Bartholomew, Debashish Behera, Sumit Bhatia, Sanjay Bindra, Aminah Bliss, Dave Brinton, Julianne Brown, Alexander Brownie, Tamara Callahan, David Canes, Bryan Casey, Aaron Caughey, Hebert Chen, Jonathan Cheng, Arnold Cheung, Arnold Chin, Simion Chiosea, Yoon Cho, Samuel Chung, Gretchen Conant, Vladimir Coric, Christopher Cosgrove, Ronald Cowan, Karekin R. Cunningham, A. Sean Dalley, Rama Dandamudi, Sunit Das, Ryan Armando Dave, John David, Emmanuel de la Cruz, Robert DeMello, Navneet Dhillon, Sharmila Dissanaike, David Donson, Adolf Etchegaray, Alea Eusebio, Jose M. Fierro, Priscilla A. Frase, David Frenz, Kristin Gaumer, Yohannes Gebreegziabher, Anil Gehi, Tony George, L.M. Gotanco, Parul Goyal, Alex Grimm, Rajeev Gupta, Ahmad Halim, Sue Hall, David Hasselbacher, Tamra Heimert, Michelle Higley, Dan Hoit, Eric Jackson, Tim Jackson, Sundar Jayaraman, Pei-Ni Jone, Aarchan Joshi, Rajni K. Jutla, Faiyaz Kapadi, Seth Karp, Aaron S. Kesselheim, Sana Khan, Andrew Pin-wei Ko, Francis Kong, Paul Konitzky, Warren S. Krackov, Benjamin H.S. Lau, Ann LaCasce, Connie Lee, Scott Lee, Guillermo Lehmann, Kevin Leung, Paul Levett, Warren Levinson, Eric Ley, Ken Lin, Pavel Lobanov, J. Mark Maddox, Aram Mardian, Rinku Mehta, Samir Mehta, Gil Melmed, Joe Messina, Robert Mosca, Michael Murphy, Vivek Nandkarni, Siva Naraynan, Carvell Nguyen, Linh Nguyen, Deanna Nobleza, Craig Nodurft, George Noumi, Darin T. Okuda, Adam L. Palance, Paul Pamphrus, Jinha Park, Sonny Patel, Ricardo Pietrobon, Riva L. Rahl, Aashita Randeria, Rachan Reddy, Beatriu Reig, Marilou Reyes, Jeremy Richmon, Tai Roe, Rick Roller, Rajiv Roy, Diego Ruiz, Anthony Russell, Sanjay Sahgal, Urmimala Sarkar, John Schilling, Isabell Schmitt, Daren Schuhmacher, Sonal Shah, Edie Shen, Justin Smith, John Stulak, Lillian Su, Julie Sundaram, Rita Suri, Seth Sweetser, Antonio Talayero, Merita Tan, Mark Tanaka, Eric Taylor, Jess Thompson, Indi Trehan, Raymond Turner, Okafo Uchenna, Eric Uyguanco, Richa Varma, John Wages, Alan Wang, Eunice Wang, Andy Weiss, Amy Williams, Brian Yang, Hany Zaky, Ashraf Zaman, and David Zipf.

Please let us know if your name has been missed or misspelled and we will be happy to make the update in the next edition.

For generously contributing images to the entire Underground Clinical Vignette Step 2 series, we collectively thank the staff at Blackwell Publishing in Oxford, Boston, and Berlin as well as:

- Alfred Cuschieri, Thomas P.J. Hennessy, Roger M. Greenhalgh, David I. Rowley, Pierce A. Grace (Clinical Surgery, © 1996 Blackwell Science), Figures 13.23, 13.35b, 13.51, 15.13, 15.2.

- Berg D. Advanced Clinical Skills and Physical Diagnosis. Blackwell Science Ltd., 1999. Figures 7.10, 7.12, 7.13, 7.2, 7.3, 7.7, 7.8, 7.9, 8.1, 8.2, 8.4, 8.5, 9.2, 10.2, 11.3, 11.5, 12.6.
- John Axford (Medicine, © 1996 Blackwell Science), Figures f3.10, 2.103a, 2.110b, 3.20a, 3.20b, 3.25b, 3.38a, 5.9bi, 5.9bii, 6.41a, 6.41b, 6.74b, 6.74c, 7.78ai, 7.78aii, 7.78b, 8.47b, 9.9e, f3.17, f3.36, f3.37, f5.27, f5.28, f5.45a, f5.48, f5.49a, f5.50, f5.65a, f5.67, f5.68, f8.27a, 10.120b, 11.63b, 11.63c, 11.68a, 11.68b, 11.68c, 12.37a, 12.37b.
- Peter Armstrong, Martin L. Wastie (Diagnostic Imaging, 4th Edition, © 1998 Blackwell Science), Figures 2.100, 2.108d, 2.109, 2.11, 2.112, 2.121, 2.122, 2.13, 2.1ba, 2.1bb, 2.36, 2.53, 2.54, 2.69a, 2.71, 2.80a, 2.81b, 2.82, 2.84a, 2.84b, 2.88, 2.89a, 2.89b, 2.90b, 2.94a, 2.94b, 2.96, 2.97, 2.98a, 2.98c, 3.11, 3.19, 3.20, 3.21, 3.22, 3.28, 3.30, 3.34, 3.35b, 3.35c, 3.36, 4.7, 4.8, 4.9, 5.29, 5.33, 5.58, 5.62, 5.63, 5.64, 5.65b, 5.66a, 5.66b, 5.69, 5.71, 5.75, 5.8, 5.9, 6.17a, 6.17b, 6.25, 6.28, 6.29c, 6.30, 7.13, 7.17a, 7.45a, 7.45b, 7.46, 7.50, 7.52, 7.53a, 7.57a, 7.58, 8.7a, 8.7b, 8.7c, 8.86, 8.8a, 8.96, 8.9a, 9.17a, 9.17b, 10.13a, 10.13b, 10.14a, 10.14b, 10.14c, 10.17a, 10.17b, 11.16b, 11.17a, 11.17b, 11.19, 11.23, 11.24, 11.2b, 11.2d, 11.30a, 11.30b, 12.12, 12.15, 12.18, 12.19, 12.3, 12.4, 12.8a, 12.8b, 13.13a, 13.18, 13.18a, 13.20, 13.22a, 13.22b, 13.29, 14.14a, 14.5, 14.6a, 15.25b, 15.29b, 15.31, 15.37, 17.4.
- N.C. Hughes-Jones, S.N. Wickramasinghe (Lecture Notes On: Haematology, 6th Edition, © 1996 Blackwell Science), Figures 2.1b, 2.2a, 3.14, 3.8, 4.3, 5.2b, 5.5a, 5.8, 7.1, 7.2, 7.3, 7.5, 8.1, 10.5b, 10.6, 11.1, plate 29, plate 34, plate 44, plate 45, plate 48, plate 5, plate 42.
- Thomas Grumme, Wolfgang Kluge, Konrad Kretzschmar, Andreas Roesler (Cerebral and Spinal Computed Tomography, 3rd Edition, © 1998 Blackwell Science), Figures 16.2b, 16.3, 16.6a, 17.1a, 18.1c, 18.5, 41.3c, 41.3d, 44.3, 46.8, 47.7, 48.2, 48.6a, 53.5, 55.2a, 55.2c, 56.2b, 57.1, 61.3a, 61.3b, 63.1a, 64.3a, 65.3c, 66.3b, 67.6, 70.1a, 70.3, 81.2a, 81.4, 82.2, 82.3, 84.6.
- P.R. Patel (Lecture Notes On: Radiology, © 1998 Blackwell Science), Figures 2.15, 2.16, 2.25, 2.26, 2.30, 2.31, 2.33, 2.36, 3.11, 3.16, 3.19, 3.4, 3.7, 4.19, 4.20, 4.38, 4.44, 4.45, 4.46, 4.47, 4.49, 4.5, 5.14, 5.6, 6.18, 6.19, 6.20, 6.21, 6.22, 6.31a, 6.31b, 7.18, 7.19, 7.21, 7.22, 7.32, 7.34, 7.41, 7.46a, 7.46b, 7.48, 7.49, 7.9, 8.2, 8.3, 8.4, 8.5, 8.8, 8.9, 9.12, 9.2, 9.3, 9.8, 9.9, 10.11, 10.16, 10.5.
- Ramsay Vallance (An Atlas of Diagnostic Radiology in Gastroenterology, © 1999 Blackwell Science), Figures 1.22, 2.57, 2.27, 2.55a, 2.58, 2.59.

HOW TO USE THIS BOOK

This series was originally developed to address the increasing number of clinical vignette questions on medical examinations, including the USMLE Step 1 and Step 2.

Each UCV 2 book uses a series of approximately **50 "supra-prototypical" cases as a way to condense testable facts and associations**. The clinical vignettes in this series are designed to give added emphasis to pathogenesis, epidemiology, management, and complications. They also contain relevant extensive B/W imaging plates within each book. Additionally, each UCV 2 book contains approximately 30 to 60 MiniCases that focus on presenting only the key facts for that disease in a tightly edited fashion. Although each case tends to present all the signs, symptoms, and diagnostic findings for a particular illness, **patients generally will not present with such a "complete" picture either clinically or on a medical examination**. Cases are not meant to simulate a potential real patient or an exam vignette. **All the boldfaced "buzzwords" are for learning purposes** and are not necessarily expected to be found in any one patient with the disease.

Definitions of selected important terms are placed within the vignettes in (small caps) in parentheses. Other parenthetical remarks often refer to the pathophysiology or mechanism of disease. The format should also help students learn to present cases succinctly during oral "bullet" presentations on clinical rotations. The cases are meant to serve as a condensed review, not as a primary reference. The information provided in this book has been prepared with a great deal of thought and careful research. This book should not, however, be considered as your sole source of information. Corrections, suggestions, and submissions of new cases are encouraged and will be acknowledged and incorporated when appropriate in future editions.

We hope that you find the *Blackwell Underground Clinical Vignettes* series informative and useful. We welcome feedback and suggestions you have about this book, or any published by Blackwell Publishing.

Please e-mail us at medfeedback@bos.blackwellpublishing.com.

ABBREVIATIONS

A-a	alveolar-arterial (oxygen gradient)
AAA	abdominal aortic aneurysm
ABCs	airway, breathing, circulation
ABGs	arterial blood gases
ABPA	allergic bronchopulmonary aspergillosis
ABVD	Adriamycin, bleomycin, vinblastine, dacarbazine (chemotherapy)
ACE	angiotensin-converting enzyme
ACTH	adrenocorticotropic hormone
ADA	adenosine deaminase, American Diabetic Association
ADH	antidiuretic hormone
ADHD	attention-deficit hyperactivity disorder
AED	automatic external defibrillator
AFP	α-fetoprotein
AI	aortic insufficiency
AICD	automatic internal cardiac defibrillator
AIDS	acquired immunodeficiency syndrome
ALL	acute lymphocytic leukemia
ALS	amyotrophic lateral sclerosis
ALT	alanine aminotransferase
AML	acute myelogenous leukemia
AMP	adenosine monophosphate
ANA	antinuclear antibody
ANCA	antineutrophil cytoplasmic antibody
Angio	angiography
AP	anteroposterior
aPTT	activated partial thromboplastin time
ARDS	adult respiratory distress syndrome
ARF	acute renal failure
AS	ankylosing spondylitis
ASA	acetylsalicylic acid
5-ASA	5-aminosalicylic acid
ASD	atrial septal defect
ASO	antistreptolysin O
AST	aspartate aminotransferase
ATLS	Advanced Trauma Life Support (protocol)
ATN	acute tubular necrosis
ATPase	adenosine triphosphatase
ATRA	all-*trans*-retinoic acid
AV	arteriovenous, atrioventricular
AVPD	avoidant personality disorder
AXR	abdominal x-ray
AZT	azidothymidine (zidovudine)
BCG	bacille Calmette-Guérin
BE	barium enema
BP	blood pressure

BPD	borderline personality disorder
BPH	benign prostatic hypertrophy
BPK	B-cell progenitor kinase
BPM	beats per minute
BUN	blood urea nitrogen
CAA	cerebral amyloid angiopathy
CABG	coronary artery bypass grafting
CAD	coronary artery disease
CALLA	common acute lymphoblastic leukemia antigen
C-ANCA	cytoplasmic antineutrophil cytoplasmic antibody
CAO	chronic airway obstruction
CAP	community-acquired pneumonia
CBC	complete blood count
CBD	common bile duct
CBT	cognitive behavioral therapy
CCU	cardiac care unit
CD	cluster of differentiation
CDC	Centers for Disease Control
CEA	carcinoembryonic antigen
CF	cystic fibrosis
CFTR	cystic fibrosis transmembrane regulator
CFU	colony-forming unit
CHF	congestive heart failure
CJD	Creutzfeldt–Jakob disease
CK	creatine kinase
CK-MB	creatine kinase, MB fraction
CLL	chronic lymphocytic leukemia
CML	chronic myelogenous leukemia
CMV	cytomegalovirus
CN	cranial nerve
CNS	central nervous system
CO	cardiac output
COPD	chronic obstructive pulmonary disease
CPAP	continuous positive airway pressure
CPK	creatine phosphokinase
CPR	cardiopulmonary resuscitation
CRP	C-reactive protein
CSF	cerebrospinal fluid
CT	computed tomography
CVA	cerebrovascular accident
CXR	chest x-ray
D&C	dilatation and curettage
DAF	decay-accelerating factor
DC	direct current
DEXA	dual-energy x-ray absorptiometry

DHEA	dehydroepiandrosterone
DIC	disseminated intravascular coagulation
DIP	distal interphalangeal (joint)
DKA	diabetic ketoacidosis
DL_{CO}	diffusing capacity of carbon monoxide
DM	diabetes mellitus
DMD	Duchenne's muscular dystrophy
DNA	deoxyribonucleic acid
DNase	deoxyribonuclease
dsDNA	double-stranded DNA
DTP	diphtheria, tetanus, pertussis (vaccine)
DTRs	deep tendon reflexes
DTs	delirium tremens
DUB	dysfunctional uterine bleeding
DVT	deep venous thrombosis
EBV	Epstein–Barr virus
ECG	electrocardiography
Echo	echocardiography
ECMO	extracorporeal membrane oxygenation
EDTA	ethylenediamine tetraacetic acid
EEG	electroencephalography
EF	ejection fraction
EGD	esophagogastroduodenoscopy
E:I	expiratory-to-inspiratory (ratio)
ELISA	enzyme-linked immunosorbent assay
EM	electron microscopy
EMG	electromyography
ER	emergency room
ERCP	endoscopic retrograde cholangiopancreatography
ESR	erythrocyte sedimentation rate
EtOH	ethanol
FDA	Food and Drug Administration
Fe_{Na}	fractional excretion of sodium
FEV_1	forced expiratory volume in 1 second
FIGO	International Federation of Gynecology and Obstetrics (classification)
FIo_2	fraction of inspired oxygen
FNA	fine-needle aspiration
FRC	functional residual capacity
FSH	follicle-stimulating hormone
FTA	fluorescent treponemal antibody
FTA-ABS	fluorescent treponemal antibody absorption test
5-FU	5-fluorouracil
FVC	forced vital capacity
G6PD	glucose-6-phosphate dehydrogenase
GA	gestational age

GABA	gamma-aminobutyric acid
GABHS	group A β-hemolytic streptococcus
GAD	generalized anxiety disorder
GBM	glomerular basement membrane
G-CSF	granulocyte colony-stimulating factor
GERD	gastroesophageal reflux disease
GFR	glomerular filtration rate
GGT	gamma-glutamyltransferase
GI	gastrointestinal
GnRH	gonadotropin-releasing hormone
GU	genitourinary
HAV	hepatitis A virus
Hb	hemoglobin
HBcAg	hepatitis B core antigen
HBsAg	hepatitis B surface antigen
HBV	hepatitis B virus
hCG	human chorionic gonadotropin
HCl	hydrogen chloride
HCO_3	bicarbonate
Hct	hematocrit
HCV	hepatitis C virus
HDL	high-density lipoprotein
HEENT	head, eyes, ears, nose, and throat
HELLP	hemolysis, elevated liver enzymes, low platelets (syndrome)
HEV	hepatitis E virus
HGPRT	hypoxanthine-guanine phosphoribosyltransferase
HHV	human herpesvirus
5-HIAA	5-hydroxyindoleacetic acid
HIDA	hepato-iminodiacetic acid (scan)
HIV	human immunodeficiency virus
HLA	human leukocyte antigen
HPF	high-power field
HPI	history of present illness
HPV	human papillomavirus
HR	heart rate
HRCT	high-resolution computed tomography
HS	hereditary spherocytosis
HSG	hysterosalpingography
HSV	herpes simplex virus
HUS	hemolytic-uremic syndrome
IABC	intra-aortic balloon counterpulsation
ICA	internal carotid artery
ICD	implantable cardiac defibrillator
ICP	intracranial pressure
ICU	intensive care unit

ID/CC	identification and chief complaint
IDDM	insulin-dependent diabetes mellitus
IE	infectious endocarditis
IFA	immunofluorescent antibody
Ig	immunoglobulin
IL	interleukin
IM	infectious mononucleosis, intramuscular
INH	isoniazid
INR	International Normalized Ratio
123-ISS	iodine-123-labeled somatostatin
IUD	intrauterine device
IUGR	intrauterine growth retardation
IV	intravenous
IVC	inferior vena cava
IVIG	intravenous immunoglobulin
IVP	intravenous pyelography
JRA	juvenile rheumatoid arthritis
JVD	jugular venous distention
JVP	jugular venous pressure
KOH	potassium hydroxide
KS	Kaposi's sarcoma
KUB	kidney, ureter, bladder
LA	left atrium
LAMB	lentigines, atrial myxoma, blue nevi (syndrome)
LD	Leishman-Donovan (body)
LDH	lactate dehydrogenase
LDL	low-density lipoprotein
LES	lower esophageal sphincter
LFTs	liver function tests
LH	luteinizing hormone
LHRH	luteinizing hormone–releasing hormone
LKM	liver-kidney microsomal (antibody)
LMN	lower motor neuron
LP	lumbar puncture
L/S	lecithin-to-sphingomyelin (ratio)
LSD	lysergic acid diethylamide
LV	left ventricle, left ventricular
LVH	left ventricular hypertrophy
Lytes	electrolytes
Mammo	mammography
MAO	monoamine oxidase (inhibitor)
MAP	mean arterial pressure
MCA	middle cerebral artery
MCHC	mean corpuscular hemoglobin concentration
MCP	metacarpophalangeal (joint)

MCV	mean corpuscular volume
MDMA	3,4-methylene-dioxymethamphetamine ("Ecstasy")
MEN	multiple endocrine neoplasia
MGUS	monoclonal gammopathy of undetermined origin
MHC	major histocompatibility complex
MI	myocardial infarction
MIBG	metaiodobenzylguanidine
MMR	measles, mumps, rubella (vaccine)
MPTP	1-methyl-4-phenyl-tetrahydropyridine
MR	magnetic resonance (imaging)
mRNA	messenger ribonucleic acid
MRSA	methicillin-resistant *Staphylococcus aureus*
MS	multiple sclerosis
MTP	metatarsophalangeal (joint)
MuSK	muscle-specific kinase
MVA	motor vehicle accident
NADPH	reduced nicotinamide adenine dinucleotide phosphate
NAME	nevi, atrial myxoma, myxoid neurofibroma, ephilides (syndrome)
NG	nasogastric
NIDDM	non-insulin-dependent diabetes mellitus
NMDA	*N*-methyl-D-aspartate
NPO	nil per os (nothing by mouth)
NSAID	nonsteroidal anti-inflammatory drug
Nuc	nuclear medicine
OCD	obsessive-compulsive disorder
OCP	oral contraceptive pill
OCPD	obsessive-compulsive personality disorder
17-OHP	17-hydroxyprogesterone
OPC	organophosphate and carbamate
OS	opening snap
OTC	over the counter
PA	posteroanterior
2-PAM	pralidoxime
P-ANCA	perinuclear antineutrophil cytoplasmic antibody
Pao_2	partial pressure of oxygen
PAS	periodic acid Schiff
PBS	peripheral blood smear
Pco_2	partial pressure of carbon dioxide
PCOD	polycystic ovary disease
PCP	phencyclidine
PCR	polymerase chain reaction
PCV	polycythemia vera
PDA	patent ductus arteriosus
PE	physical exam
PEEP	positive end-expiratory pressure

PET	positron emission tomography
PFTs	pulmonary function tests
PID	pelvic inflammatory disease
PIP	proximal interphalangeal (joint)
PKU	phenylketonuria
PMI	point of maximal impulse
PMN	polymorphonuclear (leukocyte)
PO	per os (by mouth)
Po_2	partial pressure of oxygen
PPD	purified protein derivative
PROM	premature rupture of membranes
PRPP	phosphoribosyl pyrophosphate
PSA	prostate-specific antigen
PT	prothrombin time
PTE	pulmonary thromboembolism
PTH	parathyroid hormone
PTSD	post-traumatic stress disorder
PTT	partial thromboplastin time
RA	rheumatoid arthritis, right atrial
RBC	red blood cell
RDW	red-cell distribution width
REM	rapid eye movement
RF	rheumatoid factor
RhoGAM	Rh immune globulin
RNA	ribonucleic acid
RPR	rapid plasma reagin
RR	respiratory rate
RS	Reed-Sternberg (cell)
RSV	respiratory syncytial virus
RTA	renal tubular acidosis
RUQ	right upper quadrant
RV	residual volume, right ventricle, right ventricular
RVH	right ventricular hypertrophy
SA	sinoatrial
SAH	subarachnoid hemorrhage
Sao_2	oxygen saturation in arterial blood
SBE	subacute bacterial endocarditis
SBFT	small bowel follow-through
SC	subcutaneous
SCC	squamous cell carcinoma
SIADH	syndrome of inappropriate secretion of antidiuretic hormone
SIDS	sudden infant death syndrome
SLE	systemic lupus erythematosus
SMA	smooth muscle antibody
SSPE	subacute sclerosing panencephalitis

SSRI	selective serotonin reuptake inhibitor
STD	sexually transmitted disease
SZPD	schizoid personality disorder
T_3	triiodothyronine
T_4	thyroxine
TAB	therapeutic abortion
TB	tuberculosis
TBSA	total body surface area
TCA	tricyclic antidepressant
TCD	transcranial Doppler
TD	tardive dyskinesia
TENS	transcutaneous electrical nerve stimulation
TFTs	thyroid function tests
THC	*trans*-tetrahydrocannabinol
TIA	transient ischemic attack
TIBC	total iron-binding capacity
TIPS	transjugular intrahepatic portosystemic shunt
TLC	total lung capacity
TMJ	temporomandibular joint (syndrome)
TMP-SMX	trimethoprim-sulfamethoxazole
TNF	tumor necrosis factor
TNM	tumor, node, metastasis (staging)
ToRCH	*Toxoplasma*, rubella, CMV, herpes zoster
tPA	tissue plasminogen activator
TPO	thyroid peroxidase
TRAP	tartrate-resistant acid phosphatase
TRH	thyrotropin-releasing hormone
TSH	thyroid-stimulating hormone
TSS	toxic shock syndrome
TSST	toxic shock syndrome toxin
TTP	thrombotic thrombocytopenic purpura
TUBD	transurethral balloon dilatation
TUIP	transurethral incision of the prostate
TURP	transurethral resection of the prostate
UA	urinalysis
UGI	upper GI (series)
UMN	upper motor neuron
URI	upper respiratory infection
US	ultrasound
UTI	urinary tract infection
UV	ultraviolet
VCUG	voiding cystourethrogram
VDRL	Venereal Disease Research Laboratory
VF	ventricular fibrillation
VIN	vulvar intraepithelial neoplasia

VLDL	very low density lipoprotein
VMA	vanillylmandelic acid
V/Q	ventilation-perfusion (ratio)
VS	vital signs
VSD	ventricular septal defect
VT	ventricular tachycardia
vWF	von Willebrand factor
VZIG	varicella-zoster immune globulin
VZV	varicella-zoster virus
WAGR	Wilms' tumor, aniridia, ambiguous genitalia, mental retardation (syndrome)
WBC	white blood cell
WG	Wegener's granulomatosis
WPW	Wolff–Parkinson–White (syndrome)
XR	x-ray

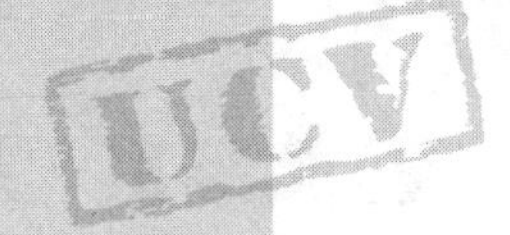

CASE 1

ID/CC A 28-year-old recently married woman complains of an **offensive vaginal discharge**.

HPI She states that the discharge is **thin, white, and foul-smelling**. She reports no vulvar pruritus or soreness.

PE VS: no fever. PE: speculum exam reveals homogenous, grayish-white, watery discharge that yields a "**fishy**" **odor** (due to volatile amines) **upon mixing with KOH** (POSITIVE "WHIFF" TEST).

Labs Vaginal **pH > 4.5**; saline smear reveals characteristic "**clue cells**" (squamous epithelial cells with stippled borders due to adherent bacteria). UA: normal.

Pathogenesis Bacterial vaginosis occurs when normal *Lactobacillus* in the vagina is **replaced by high concentrations of anaerobic bacteria**, including ***Bacteroides, Peptostreptococcus*, and *Mobiluncus* species.** ***Gardnerella vaginalis***, now recognized as normal vaginal flora, is found in increased concentrations in 90% of cases.

Management Treat with a 7-day course of **metronidazole**. Clindamycin is also effective. Treatment can be offered during pregnancy (metronidazole is contraindicated during the first trimester; topical clindamycin is contraindicated during the third trimester due to risk of premature delivery). Treatment of sexual partners is not indicated. Women with recurrent or persistent bacterial vaginosis should be screened for STDs.

Complications Increases the risks of PID, chorioamnionitis, preterm labor, premature rupture of membranes, and postpartum endometritis. Patients taking metronidazole should not drink alcohol, as it leads to a disulfiram-like reaction.

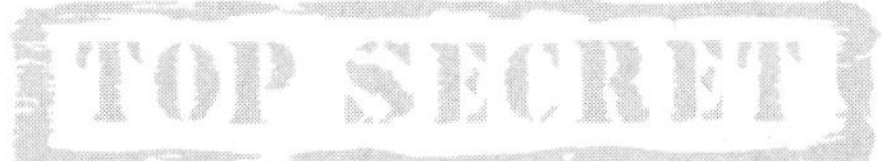

CASE 2

ID/CC A **40-year-old** woman complains of **blood-stained discharge** from the left nipple; she is concerned that she may have breast cancer.

HPI She reports a **small lump beneath the areola** of her left breast. She has **no other lumps in her breasts** or axillae and no family history of breast cancer.

PE VS: normal. PE: **serosanguineous discharge** from left nipple **and small cystic** swelling beneath areola; **no nipple retraction**; no other breast lumps or axillary lymphadenopathy; right breast normal.

Labs Tissue removed after microdochectomy reveals intraductal papilloma with ductal epithelium proliferation by histology. Cytology of nipple discharge is neither cost-effective nor reliable, since the risk of malignancy is so low.

Imaging Mammo: mass or calcification with no other pathology.

Pathogenesis Intraductal papilloma is **the most common cause of unilateral blood-stained discharge from the nipple**. Although generally a **single papilloma** in a lactiferous duct, multiple benign lesions may occur. Spontaneous clear, watery, or serosanguineous nipple discharge from a single duct has less than a 7% chance of being malignant.

Epidemiology The condition is **rare before the age of 25** and usually occurs in women between the **ages of 35 and 50**.

Management **Microdochectomy** is the preferred treatment; however, if the duct of origin of nipple bleeding cannot be identified or when bleeding is occurring from many ducts, ductogram may be done. If inconclusive, then consider **cone excision** of the major duct system.

TOP SECRET

CASE 3

GYNECOLOGY

ID/CC A **56-year-old obese** female is seen with complaints of a nonpainful **lump** in **her left breast** that she detected during routine self-examination.

HPI Her **mother died of breast cancer** at 56, and her **sister** also has the disease. The patient had an **early menarche**, is **nulliparous**, and still has regular periods (**late menopause**).

PE VS: normal. PE: 2.5-cm, **fixed, hard, irregular, nontender** mass felt in **upper outer quadrant** of breast (most common site of lesions); **retraction of overlying skin and nipple** (signs of advanced disease); no nipple discharge; left axillary lymphadenopathy; no hepatomegaly or bony tenderness; no neurologic dysfunction.

Labs CBC/Lytes: normal. LFTs: normal (alkaline phosphatase increases with bone metastasis).

Imaging CXR: normal (no evidence of metastases). [**Fig. 03A**] Mammo: ill-defined **mass** with multiple pleomorphic linear and branching microcalcifications. [**Fig. 03B**] Mammo: a different case with architecture distortion and spiculation.

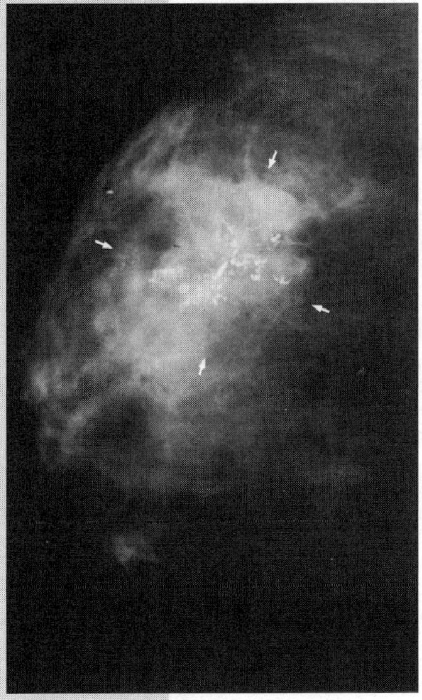

Figure 03A

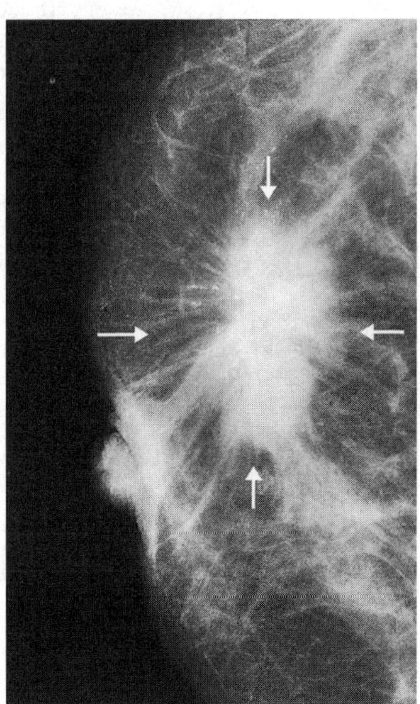

Figure 03B

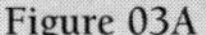

continued

CASE 3

Pathogenesis

Risk factors for breast cancer include a positive **family history, early menarche, late menopause, late first pregnancy**, nulliparity, obesity, radiation exposure, high-fat diet, geographic location (North America and Western Europe), higher socioeconomic status, atypical hyperplasia of the breast, and **breast cancer in the opposite breast**. The association between exogenous hormone use and breast cancer risk is inconclusive. Women with mutations of **tumor suppressor genes BRCA-1 or BRCA-2** are at increased risk of developing breast cancer; BRCA-1 is also associated with ovarian cancer. The inflammatory variety shows angiolymphatic spread and has an aggressive course with early, widespread metastases.

Epidemiology

In the United States, breast cancer is the **most common malignancy in females** (1 in 8 American women will develop breast cancer), followed by colorectal, lung, and endometrial cancer. The most common variety is the **infiltrating ductal type**. **Age is the single most important determinant of breast cancer incidence**, with 99% of breast carcinomas occurring after 30 years of age.

Management

A **biopsy** should be done in all cases prior to definitive treatment and should be checked for hormonal receptors. Breast-conserving surgery (LUMPECTOMY) with radiation is the preferred treatment for patients with early-stage disease; modified radical mastectomy offers no advantage over lumpectomy with axillary node dissection and radiation therapy. **Adjuvant chemotherapy** is aimed at preventing distant metastases in larger tumors and in advanced disease and usually involves cyclophosphamide, methotrexate, and fluorouracil or Adriamycin with cyclophosphamide. **Tamoxifen** may be given alone or with chemotherapy in tumors with positive estrogen receptors. Tamoxifen may also be used for breast cancer prevention in high-risk patients; drawbacks include the risk of endometrial hyperplasia and carcinoma.

Complications

Infection and/or bleeding of an exophytic tumor, distant metastases, seizures due to CNS involvement, psychological depression, and postoperative local recurrence.

CASE 4

ID/CC A 45-year-old woman complains of 2 months of recurrent **vaginal bleeding after sexual intercourse** (POSTCOITAL BLEEDING) and excessive, foul-smelling **vaginal discharge**.

HPI She has **smoked** two packs of cigarettes a day since age 22. She has been **pregnant five times, first at age 15**; she is a G5P3 TAB2. She has no history of fever, cough, urinary symptoms, nausea, vomiting, or diarrhea.

PE VS: normal. PE: **emaciated**; speculum exam reveals **ulcerated and friable cervix**; pelvic exam reveals a normal uterus and an irregular cervix that **bleeds on touch**.

Labs CBC: mild anemia; normal WBC count and differential. UA: normal. PT/PTT and INR: normal. LFTs: normal.

Imaging [**Fig. 04A**] MR, pelvis: a sagittal section shows a tumor confined to the cervix. [**Fig. 04B**] CT, pelvis: a different case in which the cervical tumor has invaded the rectum. Note the bladder (B) and rectum (R).

Pathogenesis **Human papillomavirus** (subtypes 16, 18, 33, 45, and 56), implicated in the pathogenesis of cervical cancer, is found in the transformation zone, where columnar epithelium is replaced by squamous epithelium. Most neoplastic lesions are found at the junction of the squamous and columnar epithelia (SQUAMOCOLUMNAR JUNCTION). Cervical carcinoma is staged according to the FIGO classification system as follows: 0 = in situ (INTRAEPITHELIAL CARCINOMA); I = confined to the cervix; II = extension beyond the cervix but not to the pelvic wall (A and B are without and with parametrial involvement, respectively); III = extension to the pelvic wall or to the lower vagina or the presence of hydronephrosis; IV = extension beyond the true pelvis (A and B are with spread to adjacent or distant organs, respectively). The tumor spreads primarily by local

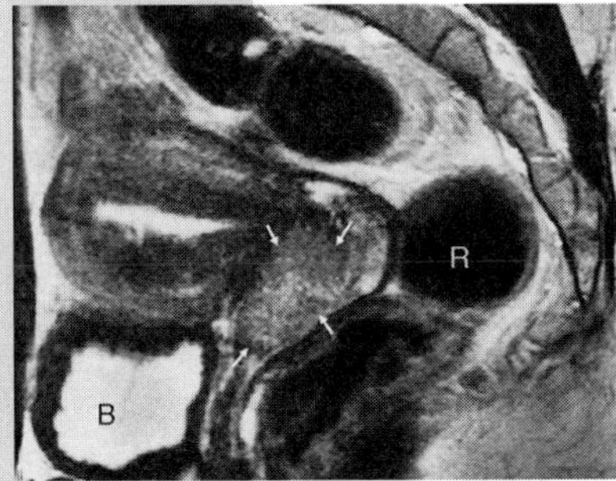

Figure 04A

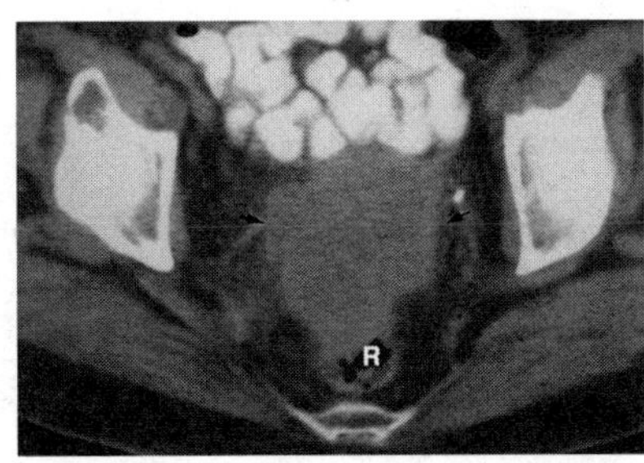

Figure 04B

continued

extension. The most common variety is **squamous cell**; less common is adenocarcinoma.

Epidemiology Cervical cancer is the **third most common malignancy of the female reproductive tract** following endometrial and ovarian cancer. It most commonly occurs in perimenopausal women. **Multiple male sexual partners, early onset of sexual activity, HPV or HIV infection**, and **smoking** are risk factors for developing cervical cancer.

Management Since the progress of the disease from dysplasia to invasive carcinoma is slow and predictable, and since clinical signs are usually present with advanced disease, emphasis should be placed on **early detection** to improve survival rates. **Pap smear** is the gold standard for screening and should be initiated with the onset of sexual activity. **Colposcopy** and **biopsy** should be considered in all suspected lesions or if a large ulcer or tumor mass is seen. No definitive treatment should be instituted without confirmation by biopsy. Cervical cancer is **staged clinically** by physical exam, CXR, cystoscopy, IVP, and proctoscopy (the last three are often replaced by CT scan). For **carcinoma in situ**, conization with surveillance is indicated for women who wish to bear children; hysterectomy is warranted if they have completed childbirth. For **stage IA**, extrafascial hysterectomy is indicated; for **stage IB and IIA** a radical hysterectomy or radiation therapy may be undertaken. For disease ranging from **stage IIB to IV**, the treatment includes radiation and chemotherapy.

Complications **Renal failure** (most common cause of death in cervical cancer) from ureteral involvement with hydroureter and hydronephrosis, **hemorrhage** (second leading cause of death), bladder and rectal fistulization, leg edema, and pelvic and back pain due to local extension.

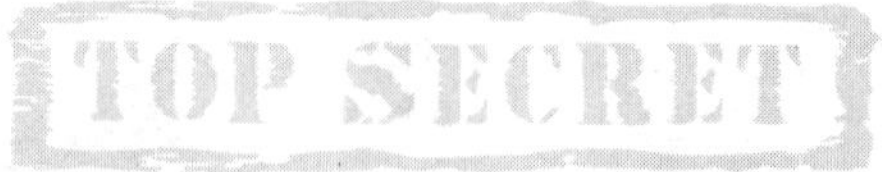

CASE 5

ID/CC A 25-year-old woman complains of **vulvar pain**, **vaginal discharge**, fever, and malaise.

HPI She was **raped** 5 days ago and has not had sexual intercourse since that time. She has no prior history of sexual intercourse.

PE VS: low-grade fever. PE: significant **tender left inguinal lymphadenopathy** (later becomes matted and forms unilocular suppurated buboes or ulcers); pelvic exam reveals heavy, foul, purulent discharge and a few **painful**, demarcated, nonindurated, **soft ulcers** (dirty, ragged edges) **with necrotic bases** in vaginal vestibule.

Labs Gram stain of pus reveals **gram-negative bacilli** arranged in characteristic "**school of fish**" pattern; culture reveals ***Haemophilus ducreyi***; Ito test (intradermal test with *H. ducreyi*) positive; darkfield illumination for treponemes negative; VDRL negative; HIV negative.

Pathogenesis Chancroid is an STD caused by the **gram-negative bacillus *H. ducreyi***. Skin trauma precedes infection (*H. ducreyi* cannot invade intact tissue).

Epidemiology Spread through direct sexual contact (with organism in an open lesion); male-to-female incidence ranges from 3:1 to 25:1. Genital ulcer diseases **enhance HIV transmission**; the association with chancroid is particularly strong.

Management The patient and the sexual partner must both be treated. In addition to **ceftriaxone**, effective drugs include **azithromycin**, **ciprofloxacin**, and **erythromycin**.

Complications Secondary infection and scarring.

CASE 6

ID/CC A 40-year-old woman presents with increasing **shortness of breath** (DYSPNEA) and **blood-tinged sputum** (HEMOPTYSIS; due to pulmonary metastases); she also complains of severe **nausea**, occasional vomiting, and **intermittent vaginal bleeding**.

HPI The patient had a dilation and vacuum aspiration (SUCTION CURETTAGE) 6 months ago for a **hydatidiform mole**.

PE VS: normal. PE: **pallor**; scattered rales in lungs; no abdominal masses; **increase in size of uterus**; no adnexal masses; speculum exam reveals **bluish-red vascular tumor**.

Labs CBC: mild anemia. LFTs: alkaline phosphatase normal. TFTs: normal. UA: normal. **Elevated serum and urinary hCG** levels.

Imaging CXR: multiple nodules (CANNONBALL METASTASES). US, pelvis: increased size of uterus, with solid echogenic material in the myometrium compatible with choriocarcinoma.

Pathogenesis Choriocarcinoma is a **highly anaplastic gestational trophoblastic malignancy** (the spectrum of the disease also includes hydatidiform mole and invasive mole) that involves the proliferation of trophoblast cells but **does not contain villi**. It may develop during or after any pregnancy (normal or abnormal). Levels of hCG should return to normal by 12 weeks after molar pregnancy evacuation; if the level plateaus or rises or if it increases in the absence of pregnancy after having returned to normal, choriocarcinoma should be strongly suspected. It invades locally and disseminates early hematogenously; the **most common sites of spread are the lungs and vagina**. Sometimes the first signs of choriocarcinoma are metastases to the external genitalia, vagina, or rectum. Stage patients according to FIGO as follows: I = confined to the uterus, II = vaginal or pelvic metastases, III = lung metastases, and IV = other distant metastases.

Epidemiology Most commonly develops after evacuation of a hydatidiform mole, although only 10% of complete molar pregnancies degenerate into malignancy. Factors associated with poor prognosis are hCG levels > 40,000, disease of > 4 months' duration, brain/liver metastases, failure of prior chemotherapy, and antecedent term pregnancy.

Management Histologic confirmation not required for treatment. **Chemotherapy** may consist of methotrexate or actinomycin D alone (in nonmetastatic disease or in metastatic disease with a good prognosis) or triple therapy with chlorambucil, actinomycin D, and methotrexate (in metastatic disease

continued

with a poor prognosis). Radiotherapy may be employed in disease involving brain or liver metastases.

Complications

Complications include CNS, liver, and kidney metastases; bone marrow aplasia with pancytopenia due to chemotherapy; oral and GI ulcers; and elevated liver enzymes. β-hCG has partial TSH activity, which may cause thyrotoxicosis.

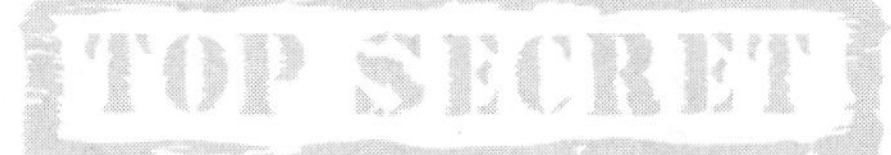

CASE 7

ID/CC A 21-year-old female complains of a **rash** on her limbs and trunk of 4 days' duration with **pain** in both **wrists and elbows**; yesterday her left **knee** became **swollen** and is now tender and "hot."

HPI She is **sexually active**. Two months ago she developed a **vaginal discharge** after several **unprotected** sexual encounters with **multiple partners**.

PE VS: **fever** (37.8°C). PE: **painful**, nonpruritic **papulovesicular rash** on an erythematous base over anterior and posterior chest and on limbs, with some **pustules on distal extremities** (ACRODERMATITIS; may also be hemorrhagic or necrotic); rash blanches with pressure; left knee **edematous, erythematous, warm** to the touch, and painful to passive and active motion with restricted range of motion; inflammation and tenderness of Achilles tendons as well as flexor tendons of both wrists (TENOSYNOVITIS).

Labs CBC: **pleocytosis** (90,000/mm^3), mostly **PMNs. Gram stain** (of cervical mucus) reveals **intracellular gram-negative diplococci**, later confirmed by **culture** in chocolate agar and Thayer-Martin medium; blood culture positive for gonococcus (positive in 50% of cases); throat swab negative; **knee joint tap** reveals abundant gonococci; RPR nonreactive.

Imaging XR, knees: effusion with soft tissue swelling; no osseous articular damage (negative in early stage, but may rapidly destroy cartilage and articular surfaces if left untreated).

Pathogenesis *Neisseria gonorrhoeae* is the causative agent of **arthritis-dermatitis syndrome**; spread from genital infection via the bloodstream (bacteremia). It is typically characterized by painful multiple joints (MIGRATORY POLYARTHRALGIA) with tenosynovitis followed by a monoarticular (usually knee) arthritis and an acral rash that is usually papulovesicular but may also be hemorrhagic or necrotic.

Epidemiology Arthritis-dermatitis syndrome occurs much **more frequently in females** and during pregnancy and menstruation; it occurs in 1% of all gonorrheal infections.

Management **Cultures** (blood, rectum, throat, synovial fluid, skin) are needed owing to the high rate of false negatives. **Antibiotics** are the mainstay of therapy; administer **ceftriaxone** or spectinomycin (for penicillin-allergic patients) with doxycycline for possible concomitant chlamydial infection (50% incidence). **RPR** is needed to rule out syphilis. Sexual relations

continued

must be strictly avoided or condoms must be used to prevent spread. It is also important to treat the partner; carriers may be asymptomatic.

Complications **PID**, **perihepatitis** (FITZ-HUGH–CURTIS SYNDROME), pelvic adhesions leading to infertility, hepatitis, meningitis, pericarditis, endocarditis, postinfectious arthritis with deformity and persistence of sterile joint effusions.

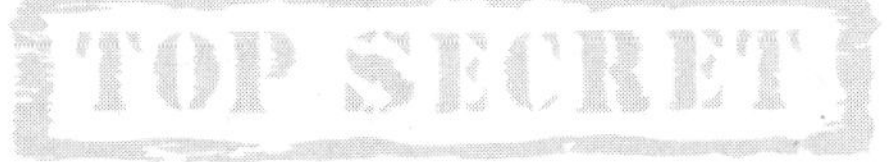

CASE 8

ID/CC A 17-year-old female is seen with complaints of **prolonged** (> 7 days) and **excessive** (> 80 mL) **menstrual bleeding** (MENORRHAGIA) and **increased menstrual frequency** (POLYMENORRHEA) for the past 6 months.

HPI The patient **denies any breast tenderness** or **lower abdominal pain** (anovulatory cycles). She is afebrile, has no vaginal discharge (making endometritis unlikely), and is not sexually active. Her menarche was at age 14.

PE VS: normal. PE: chest and abdomen normal; no thyroid enlargement; no signs of hyper- or hypothyroidism; no hyperpigmentation of hands; no leg edema; neurologic exam normal; pelvic exam reveals no masses; uterus normal size; no palpable adnexa or cervical motion tenderness.

Labs CBC: hypochromic, **microcytic anemia** (due to chronic blood loss and iron deficiency). Lytes: normal. PT/PTT: normal. UA: normal. TFTs, LH, FSH, and prolactin normal; pregnancy test negative.

Imaging CXR/KUB: normal. US, pelvis: no uterine masses; normal size; no products of conception are seen within or outside the uterus.

Pathogenesis Dysfunctional uterine bleeding (DUB) is either **anovulatory** (more common) or **ovulatory**. In anovulatory DUB, no corpus luteum develops and progesterone is absent. Unopposed estrogen results in proliferation, necrosis, and random, asynchronous shedding of the endometrium (irregular bleeding). In ovulatory DUB, the corpus luteum develops but does not secrete enough progesterone to stabilize the endometrium (LUTEAL PHASE DEFECT).

Epidemiology The most common cause of abnormal uterine bleeding. The two peaks of incidence are **puberty** and **perimenopausal years** (more common). Associated with polycystic ovary syndrome (STEIN–LEVENTHAL SYNDROME).

Management After an **underlying pathologic condition** has been ruled out, **OCPs** or **cyclical progestogens** may be given to regulate menstruation and prevent excessive bleeding on a long-term basis after acute bleeding is stopped with estrogen. D&C may be indicated for protracted or refractory bleeding. If a patient wishes to become pregnant, induction of ovulation with **clomiphene** may be contemplated. TSH and prolactin levels should be checked to rule out thyroid disease and hyperprolactinemia as causes of irregular menses. **Hysteroscopy and biopsy** are valuable adjuncts in evaluation. Any peri- or postmenopausal woman with a history of abnormal bleeding should undergo **endometrial biopsy** to rule out carcinoma.

Complications Anemia; endometrial hyperplasia with risk of carcinoma.

CASE 9

ID/CC A **61-year-old** nun presents with profuse **vaginal bleeding**.

HPI She reports some **blood loss** with passage of **large clots** a month ago. She has **no pain** but has had significant **weight loss** over the past 3 months. She is **postmenopausal**, has not had sexual intercourse for many years, and has never been pregnant. She has never had a Pap smear.

PE VS: tachycardia (HR 110); mild hypotension (BP 100/60); no fever. PE: **obese**, pale, and ill-looking; atrophic vulva; speculum exam reveals old blood in cervical canal and vagina; uterus **enlarged but mobile; no adnexal swelling**; cervix patulous; clot seen protruding from os; uterine cavity D&C confirmed a wide, expanded cavity; **necrotic tumor obtained from all surfaces; curettage provoked heavy bleeding** and patient received three units of blood.

Labs CBC: **normocytic, normochromic anemia** (blood loss). Pap smear reveals atrophic tissue; endocervical curettage reveals **no tumor**; endometrial curettage reveals poorly differentiated **adenocarcinoma** with invasion into underlying myometrium and extensive necrosis.

Imaging US, pelvis: uniformly **enlarged uterus; cavity expanded** and contained echoes consistent with blood clot and debris; no ovarian enlargement. US, transvaginal: endometrial stripe > 8 mm. [**Fig. 09**] CT, pelvis: a

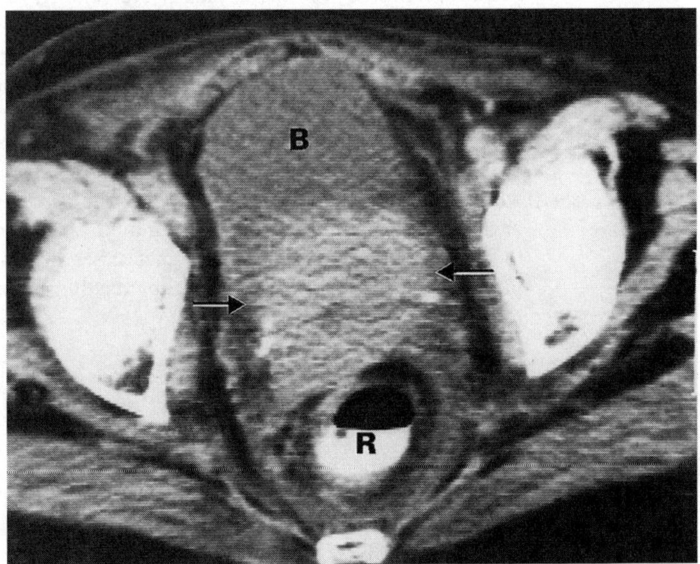

Figure 09

continued

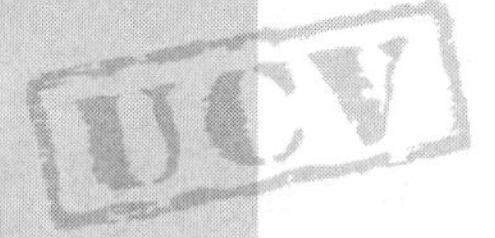

different case showing an irregular uterine mass between the bladder (B) and rectum (R).

Pathogenesis

Endometrial carcinoma is a neoplastic disease **of unknown etiology**. Most women have a history of **unopposed estrogen exposure**; however, endometrial carcinoma may develop in patients (especially older patients) without endometrial hyperplasia. Other risk factors include **obesity**, **nulliparity**, **diabetes**, hypertension, chronic tamoxifen use and **late menopause**. The tumor is spread primarily by direct extension to the cervix and myometrium through the fallopian tubes to the peritoneum and via the lymphatics to the pelvic and para-aortic lymph nodes.

Epidemiology

Endometrial carcinoma is the **most common malignancy of the female genital tract** and the fourth most common cancer in females; 1 in 50 women in the United States will develop this disease. It primarily occurs in women aged **50 to 65 years**. **Adenocarcinoma** is the most common type.

Management

Any woman with postmenopausal bleeding should be worked up with a Pap smear, endocervical curettage, and endometrial biopsy. For **stage I disease**, where cancer is limited to the corpus, a total abdominal hysterectomy and bilateral salpingo-oophorectomy or radical hysterectomy will suffice; **stage II disease**, in which the cancer has involved the corpus and the cervix, is treated with preoperative intracavitary radiotherapy followed by abdominal hysterectomy, bilateral salpingo-oophorectomy, and pelvic node dissection (this is followed by radiotherapy if the nodes are found to be involved). For **stage III disease**, in which the cancer has extended outside the uterus but not outside the true pelvis, a combination of radiotherapy and chemotherapy (with progesterone) is employed; surgery in these cases is hazardous and may be attempted after pretreatment with radiotherapy. For **stage IV**, in which the cancer has spread outside the true pelvis (to either adjacent or distant organs), progestogens and multidrug chemotherapy are used to contribute to longevity; vaginal metastases may be locally excised, pulmonary metastases are responsive to progestogen, and brain and bone metastases respond to radiotherapy.

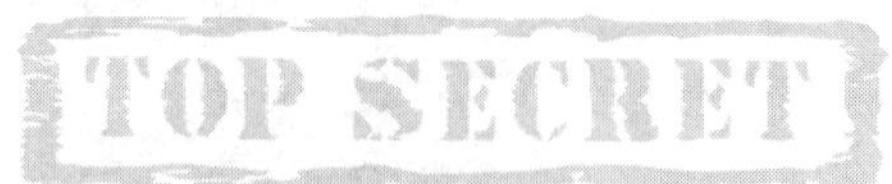

CASE 10

ID/CC A 27-year-old female complains of **inability to conceive** for 4 years.

HPI The patient has had **chronic pelvic pain** for 8 years with an **increase in the quantity and frequency of her menstrual periods** (HYPERPOLYMENORRHEA) and frequent spotting. She has also experienced progressively worsening **dysmenorrhea** and **pain during coitus** (DYSPAREUNIA).

PE VS: mild hypotension (BP 100/60); no fever. PE: umbilical area shows 3-mm **hyperpigmented, raised, nontender nodule** (extrapelvic endometrial implant); pelvic exam reveals **fixed, retroverted uterus** with **tender nodularity in uterosacral ligament**; cervix normal; **diagnostic laparoscopy** reveals multiple rust-colored ("POWDER BURN") endometrial implants in ovaries, round and broad ligaments, tubes, and cul-de-sac with adhesions.

Labs CBC/Lytes: normal. TFTs: normal. UA: normal. Infertility panel normal in patient and spouse; biopsies (of endometrial implants) reveal **stroma and glands** identical to endometrium (diagnostic of endometriosis).

Imaging CXR: normal. US, abdomen: cystic masses in both ovaries.

Pathogenesis Endometriosis is **abnormal implantation of endometrial tissue** outside the uterine cavity, leading to infertility, dyspareunia, and dysmenorrhea. Endometriomas (CHOCOLATE CYSTS) may also be seen, as may hematuria with bladder involvement or rectal bleeding with rectal involvement. It most commonly affects the **ovaries bilaterally**. The diagnosis can be made only by visual inspection of the abdomen (laparoscopy or laparotomy).

Epidemiology Mean age of presentation is 27, but incidence is not linked to age, race, or socioeconomic status. If present in older children or teens, it can be due to a defect in müllerian duct development. A **family history** of the disease, **retrograde menstruation**, and a history of **prolonged hyperpolymenorrhea** have all been associated with an increased risk of developing symptomatic endometriosis. Approximately 10% of women will develop endometriosis.

Management The first line of treatment is usually NSAIDs in conjunction with **OCPs** given in a continuous fashion (i.e., no placebo pills are taken) to suppress stimulation and growth of endometrial implants. More aggressive endometriosis may be managed with Depo-Provera (IM progesterone), Lupron (a GnRH analog), or danazol (an androgen derivative). **Surgical measures** include laparoscopic coagulation, laser ablation of lesions, or open surgery with removal of lesions and freeing of adhesions. In cases involving chronic pain that is refractory to medical treatment or when

continued

child bearing is complete, a **total hysterectomy with bilateral salpingo-oophorectomy** may be indicated. In some patients, a **medical and surgical** approach is needed for long-term pain relief.

Complications Disabling pain, infertility that is refractory to treatment, and recurrent disease when an ovary is preserved after hysterectomy.

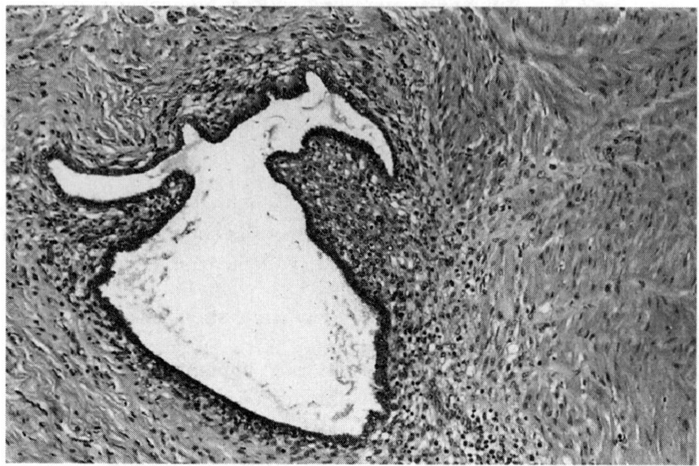

Figure 10 Island of ectopic endometrial gland and stroma within the wall of the urinary bladder.

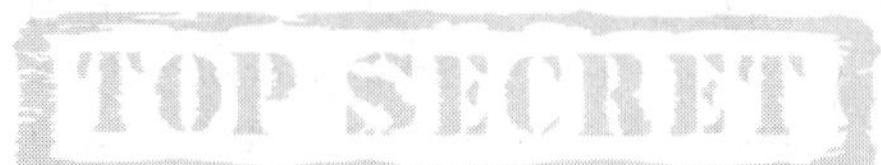

CASE 11

GYNECOLOGY

ID/CC A 22-year-old female presents after recently noticing two nonpainful "**bumps**" on her **vulva and perineum**.

HPI She denies any vaginal discharge, vulvar pruritus, burning, dysuria, or hematuria. She is **sexually active** with **multiple partners** and does not use any form of birth control.

PE PE: soft, pink, pedunculated growths 2 mm in diameter.

Labs CBC: normal. RPR nonreactive; cultures for gonorrhea and chlamydia negative; Tzanck smear negative for HSV; vaginal wet mount and KOH negative; **diagnostic biopsy** reveals papillomatous elongation and parakeratosis with cytoplasmic vacuolization (**koilocytes** are common in HPV infection).

Imaging CXR/KUB: normal.

Pathogenesis There are more than 80 different subtypes **of human papillomavirus**. Condylomata acuminata are most frequently associated with **subtypes 6 and 11**, which have little or no risk of causing neoplasia. **Subtypes 16 and 18** are associated with premalignant or malignant lesions, including cervical, vulvar, vaginal, perianal, penile, and bladder cancer. The virus is transmitted by vaginal and anal **intercourse**. Risk factors include **immunosuppression, diabetes, pregnancy, multiple sexual partners**, and **preexisting vaginitis** (HPV may colonize moist skin).

Epidemiology HPV is the most common sexually transmitted virus.

Management Always obtain a **Pap smear**. Urethroscopy may be needed in males with urethral lesions. For small warts, 25% **podophyllin** may be applied locally (contraindicated during pregnancy). Other options include the application of **trichloroacetic acid**, imiquimod, freezing with **liquid nitrogen, laser** removal, **electrocautery**, and **surgery**; 5-FU and interferon have been used with mixed results. Circumcision may help prevent recurrences in men and their partners. If there is any doubt about the diagnosis or if the lesions do not respond to therapy, an excisional biopsy should be performed to rule out malignancy.

Complications If left untreated, lesions may become large, necessitating surgical resection. Cervical lesions require monitoring via routine Pap smears and/or colposcopy for **cervical neoplasia** (although warts do not predispose to dysplasia, coinfection with HPV subtypes associated with dysplasia is common).

CASE 12

ID/CC

An 18-year-old G1P0 at 20 weeks' gestation presents with **irregular vaginal bleeding** and **mild abdominal pain**.

HPI

She also complains of **excessive nausea and vomiting** (hyperemesis), anxiety, tremulousness (hyperthyroid features), and swelling of her hands, face, and feet. A home **pregnancy test was positive**. She has been **amenorrheic for 20 weeks** but has not felt any **fetal movements**; she has at times noted the passage of grape-shaped **vesicles** vaginally. This is her first pregnancy; she denies having attempted an abortion.

PE

VS: **hypertension** (BP 145/90); **tachycardia** (HR 105). PE: appears pale and ill; bilateral pitting pedal edema present; fine tremor of hands; abdominal exam reveals that **fundal height** (24 weeks) **is more than expected** (20 weeks); uterus feels doughy in consistency (due to absence of amniotic fluid); **fetal heart not heard with Doppler**.

Labs

CBC: normocytic, normochromic anemia. UA: proteinuria. Elevated T_3 and T_4; **serum β-hCG extremely high** (> 100,000 mU/mL) relative to the expected value; **serum human placental lactogen very low**; histopathologic exam of tissue obtained after uterine evacuation reveals 1 to 2 L of a **stringy mass of swollen villi without fetal parts**; microscopy reveals **hydropic villi without blood vessels and a minor trophoblast component** (more trophoblastic tissue indicates invasive mole).

Imaging

US, pelvis: **"snowstorm" appearance** in the uterus and absence of fetal shadow; presence of bilateral **theca-lutein cysts** in the ovaries. XR, chest (done to rule out any metastases): normal.

Pathogenesis

Complete moles (46,XX) contain no fetal parts, are paternally derived, are associated with symptoms of preeclampsia, hyperemesis, and thyrotoxicosis, and have a **high potential to become invasive or to develop into a choriocarcinoma. Partial moles** (69,XXY; 69,XYY) contain fetal parts, are maternally and paternally derived, and have a **low malignant potential**. A previous molar pregnancy places the patient at higher risk for future molar pregnancies.

Epidemiology

Gestational trophoblastic neoplasia is a spectrum of disorders involving the abnormal proliferation of trophoblastic (PLACENTAL) tissue. This includes hydatidiform moles (80%), invasive moles (10% to 15%), choriocarcinoma (2% to 5%), and placental-site trophoblastic tumor (rare). In the United States, the incidence of molar pregnancy is 1 in 1,000 pregnancies. More common in women under 20 and over 40 years of age. Invasive disease develops in 10% of cases; choriocarcinoma develops in 2% of moles.

continued

Management **Immediate removal** of uterine contents by **suction evacuation and curettage.** If **follow up hCG levels do not fall, then suspect development of invasive mole or choriocarcinoma**. Pelvic exam for any cervical/vaginal metastases and regression of ovarian cysts, chest x-ray to identify pulmonary metastases, and diagnostic curettage if bleeding persists. **Pregnancy is discouraged** for 1 year during the follow-up period to prevent interference with diagnostic assaying of hCG levels. Treatment of **nonmetastatic disease consists of single-agent chemotherapy** using either methotrexate or actinomycin D; treatment of **metastatic disease** involves use of either **single-agent or multiple-agent regimens** (methotrexate, actinomycin D, chlorambucil), depending on the prognosis. Malignant forms of the disease (both invasive moles and choriocarcinoma) are exquisitely sensitive to chemotherapy. Radiotherapy may be used for brain and liver metastases. **Hysterectomy** is an option in women who have completed childbearing.

Complications Metastatic disease involving lung, liver, and brain.

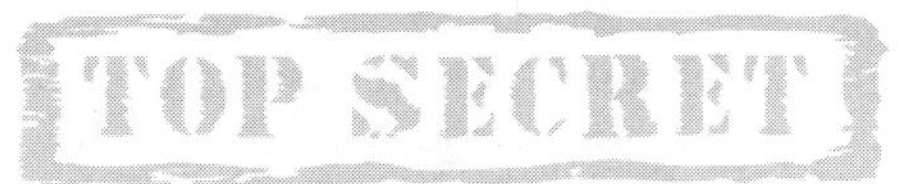

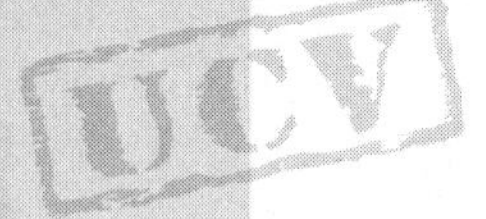

CASE 13

ID/CC A 32-year-old female is referred to a clinic for **inability to conceive**.

HPI The patient was married 2 years ago, has not used any form of contraception, and has had unprotected sexual intercourse at least twice a week. She had a therapeutic **abortion 7 years ago** and has noted **irregular bleeding** since that time. She denies any other medical or surgical history.

PE VS: normal. PE: thyroid not palpable; no breast masses, retractions, or secretion from nipple; abdomen soft and nontender; uterus not palpable; no skin rashes (rules out lupus); pelvic exam reveals uterus of normal size with regular surface, no masses, and no pain on cervical motion; adnexa not palpable; cervix appears normal; normal visual fields (decreases likelihood of pituitary involvement).

Labs CBC/Lytes/UA: normal. TFTs: normal; cortisol, prolactin, testosterone, and DHEA levels normal.

Imaging CXR/KUB: normal. US, abdomen and pelvis: intrauterine adhesions between the two inner walls of the endometrial cavity; no adnexal masses. HSG: intrauterine synechiae and patent fallopian tubes.

Pathogenesis Infertility is defined as the **inability to conceive for 1 year after regular unprotected sexual intercourse**. The most common causes of infertility are **lack of normal spermatogenesis**, **lack of ovulatory cycles**, and **anatomic defects** of the female genitalia. Causes of **male infertility** include mumps orchitis with atrophy, antisperm antibodies, Klinefelter's syndrome, retrograde ejaculation, varicocele, hypogonadotropic hypogonadism, and Sertoli-cell-only syndrome. **Female anatomic abnormalities** involved include congenital defects; acquired defects such as **Asherman's syndrome**, which consists of intrauterine adhesions (SYNECHIAE) due to previous vigorous curettage of the uterus; **PID**, which produces adhesions that may obstruct the fallopian tubes; **leiomyomata**; and **endometriosis**.

Epidemiology Infertility affects 15% of married couples with wives of childbearing age. In 10% of cases, infertility is idiopathic.

Management Measure luteal phase **progesterone levels** and **basal body temperature** (shows a biphasic curve in women who ovulate, with a peak temperature seen in consonance with the rise in progesterone following LH surge; during menstruation, temperature goes back down) to ascertain ovulation. Patients who complain of fullness of the breasts and lower abdominal/back discomfort and who have regular menstrual cycles are more likely to have regular ovulatory cycles. **Endometrial biopsy** and

continued

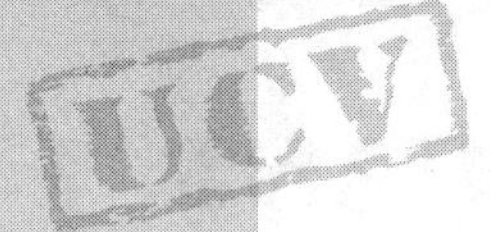

urine LH levels similarly aid in diagnosing luteal phase defects and ovulation, respectively. **Hysterosalpingography** can show the endometrial cavity and tubes, and **laparoscopy** is very helpful in diagnosing endometriosis and adhesion formation. Normal **semen analysis** (sample taken after 48 hours of abstinence) shows a volume of more than 3 mL, with a minimum of 20 million sperm/mL; normal motility entails 50% of sperm with forward motion. More than 60% of sperm should be morphologically normal, and there must be < 1 million WBCs/mL. More than 75% of infertile couples eventually conceive with treatment. Treatment varies according to the cause and ranges from induction of ovulation with **clomiphene** or gonadotropins to surgical correction of anatomic abnormalities, in vitro fertilization, and artificial insemination.

Complications

Depression, **anxiety**, disruption of family life, and multiple-gestation pregnancies after induction of ovulation.

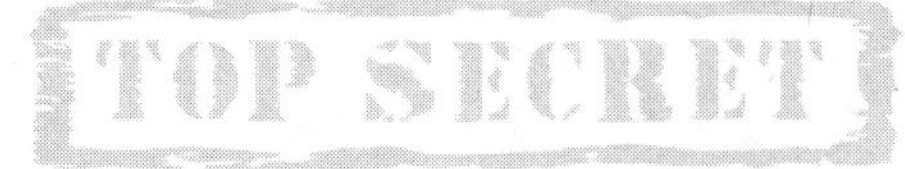

CASE 14

ID/CC A **51-year-old** woman complains of **hot flashes, night sweats, emotional lability**, depression, sleep disturbance, and inability to concentrate.

HPI She also notes **decreased libido, painful coitus** (DYSPAREUNIA) due to decreased vaginal lubrication, and **painful micturition** (DYSURIA). Her last menstrual period was six months ago.

PE Gynecologic exam reveals **atrophic vaginitis**.

Labs **Elevated FSH and LH; cholesterol and triglycerides increased** in relation to premenopausal levels (decreased HDL and increased LDL and VLDL).

Imaging CXR, spine: decreased bone density. DEXA: **osteoporosis**.

Pathogenesis Menopause is the cessation of menstrual periods due to a decline in estrogen and progesterone production from the ovaries. The peripheral conversion of adrenal androstenedione to estrogen becomes the principal source of estrogen after menopause.

Epidemiology The average age of menopause in Western societies is **51 years**.

Management **Estrogen-progesterone therapy** in women in whom the uterus is still present; give unopposed continuous estrogen therapy in women who have had a hysterectomy (**unopposed estrogen therapy increases the risk of endometrial cancer** by inducing atypical adenomatous hyperplasia). Hormone replacement should be instituted at the lowest possible doses and for the shortest period of time. **Calcium supplementation** and weight-bearing exercises should be prescribed for prevention of osteoporosis.

Complications **Atrophic vulvovaginitis, atrophic trigonitis (bladder) and urethritis, ischemic heart disease** (due to an unfavorable lipid profile), pelvic relaxation, and **osteoporosis**.

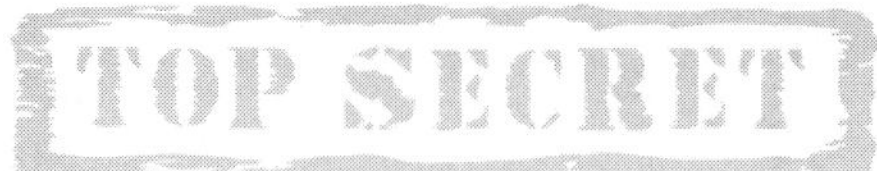

CASE 15

GYNECOLOGY

ID/CC A **38-year-old** woman presents with **left-sided weakness** and **numbness**.

HPI She is **hypertensive, obese**, and a **chronic smoker** who occasionally has **migraines**; she has been **taking OCPs** for approximately 4 years.

PE VS: hypertension (BP 145/90). PE: pupils equal, round, and reactive to light and accommodation; cranial nerves intact; left arm and leg show **2/5 strength, increased tone, and exaggerated reflexes; decreased pain sensation** on left side.

Labs CBC: increased hematocrit and hemoglobin (chronic smoker). **Cholesterol and triglycerides** markedly increased.

Imaging CT, head: **right-sided infarct**; no areas of hemorrhage.

Pathogenesis **Cerebrovascular accidents** (CVAs), **DVT**, and **pulmonary embolism** are more common in OCP users than in nonusers. This may be due to intimal and medial vascular injury, increased platelet aggregation, and a decrease in antithrombin III activity and plasminogen activator caused by the estrogen component of the pill. The effect is dose dependent; with reduction in the estrogen content of the pill, the incidence of thromboembolic disorders falls.

Epidemiology Other predisposing factors include **age > 35 years, blood group other than O**, heavy **smoking, hypertension, diabetes**, migraine, and **hyperlipidemia**.

Management Discontinue OCPs. **Heparinize** after ruling out bleeding with head CT and fecal occult blood. **Fluid restriction** and corticosteroids to prevent cerebral edema. Long-term **physiotherapy**. Where applicable, counsel the patient to stop smoking.

Complications Side effects of birth control pill use (related mainly to the estrogen component) include **thromboembolic phenomena, vaginal spotting, depression**, breast engorgement, hypertension, hepatic adenomas, nausea, weight gain, cholestasis, amenorrhea or hypomenorrhea, and decreased glucose tolerance. OCPs are contraindicated in women who are older than 35 years and smoke more than 15 cigarettes a day; those who have a history of thromboembolic disease; those who have concurrent breast, liver, or endometrial cancer; and those who have completed a term pregnancy within 10 to 14 days.

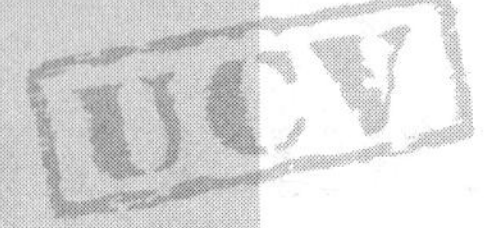

CASE 16

ID/CC A **58-year-old** woman is found to have a **pelvic mass** during a routine yearly physical examination.

HPI She is diabetic and hypertensive and has been complaining of **vague GI symptoms**, including diarrhea alternating with constipation. She has recently been feeling **lower abdominal heaviness** and notes **increasing abdominal girth**. She denies any postmenopausal bleeding or weight loss.

PE VS: normal. PE: no acute distress; abdomen firm and nontender; ascites present; **mass felt** in left iliac fossa (in postmenopausal women, regarded as **malignant until proven otherwise**); no peritoneal signs; pelvic examination confirms **left fixed, nontender, irregular solid adnexal mass**; cervix normal; rectal exam normal.

Labs CBC: mild anemia; no leukocytosis. Lytes: normal. **CA-125 elevated** (also elevated in endometriosis, fibroids, and PID). LFTs: normal. Blood glucose normal. UA: normal.

Imaging CXR: normal. CT/US, pelvis: cystic mass 6 cm in diameter with solid areas in the left ovary; omental caking; ascites.

Pathogenesis Ovarian carcinoma often attains considerable size before it is detected; nearly 75% of cases have **metastases at diagnosis**. Of all ovarian cancers, **90% are epithelial in origin**. Of these, the most common variety is **serous cystadenocarcinoma** (may also be mucinous); other types include solid endometrioid carcinomas and Brenner's tumors. Twenty percent of ovarian cancers are derived from the germ cell of the ovary (e.g., teratomas, dysgerminomas); 10% originate from the ovarian stroma (e.g., fibromas, granulosa-theca cell tumors). **Ovarian cancer is staged surgically**; according to FIGO staging, **stage I** is confined to the ovaries, **stage II** involves pelvic extension, **stage III** involves intraperitoneal and lymph node metastases, and **stage IV** shows distant metastases. Ovarian carcinoma spreads **lymphatically** to the regional nodes **directly** through peritoneal seeding and **hematogenously** to the **liver**, **bone**, and **lungs**. Carcinoma of the ovary is not always primary; metastases from the stomach (KRUKENBERG TUMOR), breast, and colon are seen in 5% to 10% of cases.

Epidemiology Ovarian cancer is the **second most common cancer** of the female reproductive tract and the **leading cause of death from gynecologic cancer** in the United States, showing an overall 5-year survival rate of about 15%. Its highest incidence is in women between the **ages of 40 and 65**. A **family history** of ovarian cancer, **nulliparity**, **delayed childbirth**, and **late age at menopause** are strong predisposing factors. OCPs have been shown to decrease the risk of ovarian cancer. Women with breast cancer have a twofold increase in ovarian cancer.

continued

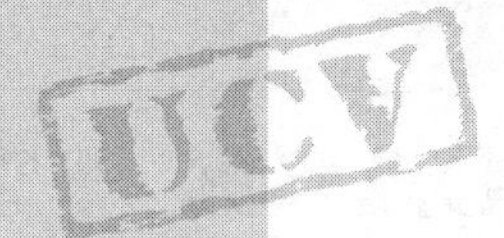

CASE 16

Management Peritoneal washings, para-aortic nodes, diaphragmatic biopsy, and omentum are taken as specimens for staging purposes at the time of the first surgical exploration. **Total abdominal hysterectomy** with **bilateral salpingo-oophorectomy**, omentectomy, and lymphadenectomy if the tumor is in its early stages. If resection is not possible, an attempt is made to **debulk** the tumor so that the remaining lesion is < 2 cm. **Chemotherapy** (platinum-based chemotherapy and taxol) and/or **radiotherapy** may then be employed with a second-look laparotomy or laparoscopy at a later date.

Complications Ascites, pelvic pain, anemia, wasting, distant metastases, and recurrence.

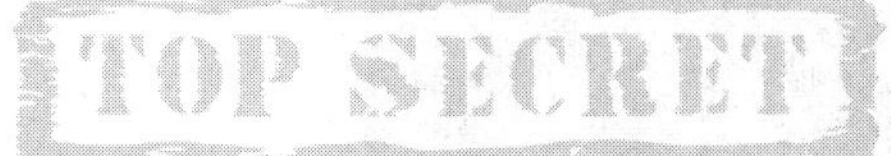

CASE 17

ID/CC

A **32-year-old** female complains of **menstrual irregularities** and a feeling of **lower abdominal pressure** of 4 months' duration.

HPI

She is nulliparous and has never used any contraception. Her last menstrual period was 1 week ago.

PE

VS: normal. PE: well hydrated, thin, and in no acute distress; soft, **rounded, nontender right lower quadrant mass**; bimanual palpation confirms **enlarged right adnexa** with freely **mobile** 7-cm mass located anterior to broad ligament; cervix appears normal.

Labs

CBC/Lytes: normal. TFTs, PT/PTT, and INR: normal. UA: normal. Pregnancy test negative.

Imaging

[**Fig. 17A**] CT, pelvis: an oval-shaped mass (1) with the same density as fat is seen posterior to the bladder (B) and has an area of hyperdensity (arrow) within. [**Fig. 17B**] XR, pelvis: another case demonstrates teeth within the cyst. [**Fig. 17C**] US, pelvis: another case shows a mixed cystic (1) and solid (2) mass with areas of calcification (3) due to teeth inside the cyst.

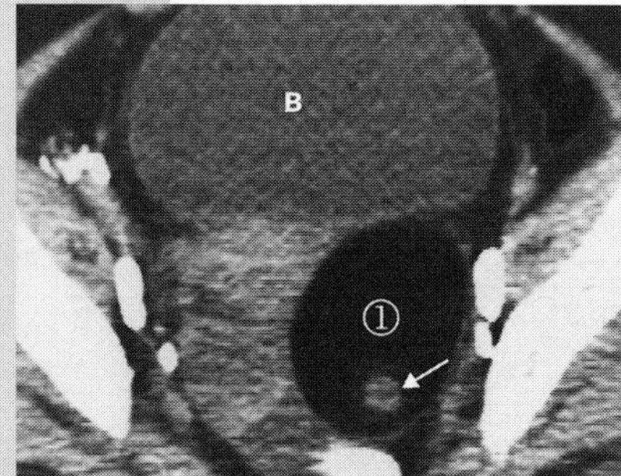

Figure 17A

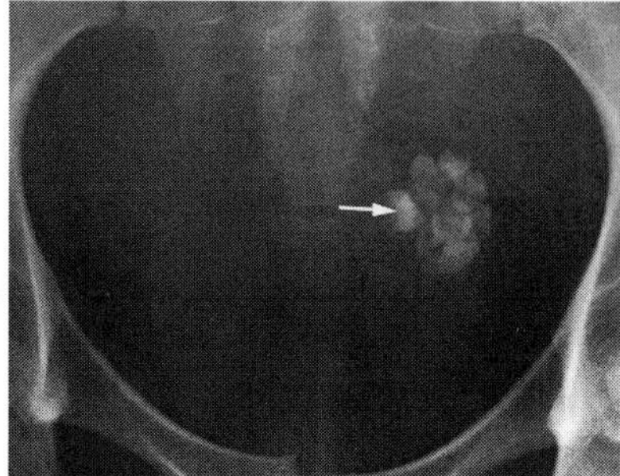
Figure 17B

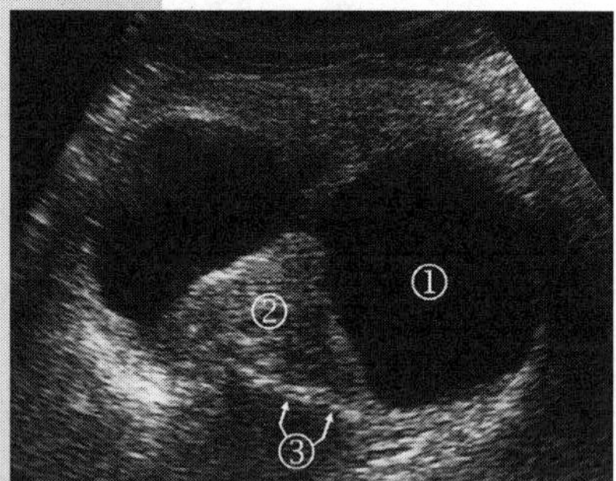

Figure 17C

continued

CASE 17

GYNECOLOGY

Pathogenesis

Mature cystic teratomas are germ cell tumors derived from ectodermal differentiation of totipotential cells and are usually benign. They may contain hair, cartilage, thyroid, nervous tissue, teeth, and skin (three germ cell layers: ectoderm, mesoderm, and endoderm) and may attain a size of up to 20 cm. When the ectodermal component is prominent, it is termed a dermoid cyst; the most common ovarian tumor in children.

Epidemiology

Comprise one-quarter of all ovarian tumors. Bilateral in 15% of cases; affect females in their third and fourth decades of life.

Management

Surgical removal of the cyst, leaving a portion of uninvolved ovary if any. Explore the contralateral ovary in view of the risk of bilaterality. Recurrence is rare.

Complications

Torsion, rupture with peritonitis, hyperthyroidism caused by secretion of thyroid hormone by ectopic colloid thyroid tissue in the ovary (STRUMA OVARII), secretion of serotonin (CARCINOID SYNDROME), and malignant transformation in a small fraction of cases (squamous cell carcinoma).

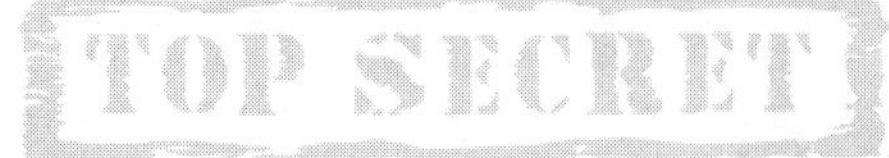

CASE 18

ID/CC A **24-year-old** woman complains of several weeks of crampy, bilateral **lower abdominal pain worsened by menses**; thick, **greenish-yellow vaginal discharge**; and vulvar irritation. This morning she woke up with increased pain, **fever, and vomiting**.

HPI She has had **unprotected sex** with **multiple sexual partners**. She has had an **IUD** since age 20.

PE VS: **fever** (39°C); hypotension (BP 85/60); tachycardia (HR 110). PE: abdomen soft; hypogastric tenderness; no masses palpable; **voluntary guarding but no rigidity**; no rebound tenderness or change in bowel sounds; pelvic exam reveals **exquisite tenderness when cervix is moved** laterally (CERVICAL MOTION TENDERNESS); **adnexa tender; abundant purulent discharge from cervical os**.

Labs CBC: **leukocytosis** (16,000) with left shift. **Elevated ESR and CRP**; Gram stain (of purulent discharge) reveals **intracellular gram-negative diplococci** (suggestive of gonorrhea) as well as increased WBCs (18 leukocytes per HPF, suggestive of chlamydia); RPR nonreactive; blood culture shows no growth at 24 hours.

Imaging US, pelvis: no masses in adnexa; enlarged, tender fallopian tubes.

Pathogenesis Pelvic inflammatory disease (PID) refers to ascending genital infection involving the endometrium, fallopian tubes, and broad ligaments (ENDOMETRITIS, SALPINGITIS, PARAMETRITIS). It is usually transmitted **sexually** via cervical infection with upward spread to the fallopian tubes. PID is typically a polymicrobial infection, but 60% to 70% of the time ***Chlamydia trachomatis*** and/or ***Neisseria gonorrhoeae*** will infect the cervical canal, damaging the protective layer and forming adhesions and fibrosis. *Bacteroides* species, *Escherichia coli, Haemophilus influenzae, Mycoplasma*, and, less commonly, tuberculosis (hematogenous route) may also be involved.

Epidemiology Incidence is highest among young females with **multiple sexual partners; unprotected sex** greatly increases the risk of developing PID. Frequent **douching**, young age, low socioeconomic status, IUD use, and **smoking** are also associated with an increased risk of developing PID. OCPs appear to have a protective effect against chlamydial PID (by thickening cervical mucus).

Management Samples of cervical exudate (consider rectal, urethral, and throat swabs) are taken. Antibiotics are then started before results are obtained. **Ceftriaxone** or **cefoxitin** plus **probenecid** followed by **doxycycline** for 14 days is the usual outpatient regimen. For inpatients, **cefoxitin** or **cefotetan** plus **doxycycline** is used. **Clindamycin plus gentamicin** is an

continued

alternative inpatient regimen. If complications such as abscess formation or peritonitis ensue, surgical drainage may be required. Indications for hospitalization include tubo-ovarian abscess, association with an IUD, patient noncompliance, signs of systemic infection, and inability to take or absorb oral antibiotics. Refer sexual partners for treatment.

Complications Infectivity (related to chronicity and recurrence), **infertility**, thickening of the tubal wall (INTERSTITIAL SALPINGITIS), hydrosalpinx, perioophoritis, **tubo-ovarian abscess** formation, perforation with generalized peritonitis, dyspareunia, ectopic pregnancy, gonococcal perihepatitis (FITZ–HUGH–CURTIS SYNDROME), intestinal obstruction due to adhesions, suppurative arthritis, and **chronic pelvic pain**.

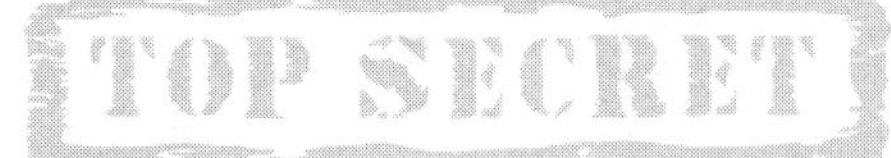

CASE 19

ID/CC A **20-year-old** woman complains **of inability to conceive, excessive menstrual flow, and bilateral lower abdominal pain.**

HPI She was treated for **pulmonary tuberculosis** a few years ago and has been unable to conceive for the past 2 years. Semen analysis of her husband is normal.

PE VS: normal HR; normal BP; low-grade fever. PE: **small, fixed adnexal masses** that are **matted and fixed to uterus** ("FROZEN PELVIS"); uterine tenderness; thickening of broad ligament.

Labs CBC: anemia. **Elevated ESR**; culture of endometrial curettage reveals ***Mycobacterium tuberculosis***; histologic examination of curettage shows presence of characteristic **granulomas; Mantoux test strongly positive**; ELISA for TB positive.

Imaging XR, chest: **cystic cavities and fibrosis** in upper lobes (old healed pulmonary tuberculosis). Hysterosalpingography (HSG) is contraindicated in a proven case of tuberculosis.

Pathogenesis Pelvic tuberculosis usually occurs when a primary lung infection invades the pelvis hematogenously. The **fallopian tube** is the most frequently involved part of the genital tract.

Epidemiology Incidence peaks in early 20s. May follow IUD insertion, hysterosalpingography, and D&C.

Management **Four-drug therapy** with INH, pyrazinamide, ethambutol, and rifampin for 2 months; continue INH and rifampin for another 6 months. **Indications for surgery** include disease progression or persistence despite antibiotic therapy; **90% of cases are cured** with intensive therapy, but **only 10% regain fertility**.

Complications Complications include INH-induced **pyridoxine deficiency** (administer pyridoxine) and **hepatotoxicity** resulting from rifampin and INH (obtain baseline LFTs). **Adhesions** within the uterine cavity form synechiae (ASHERMAN'S SYNDROME).

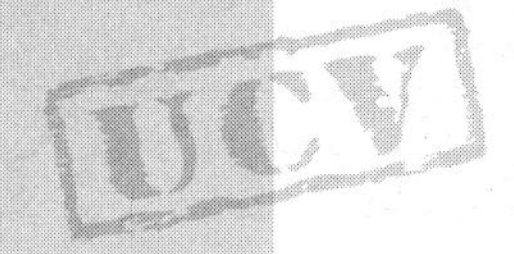

CASE 20

ID/CC A **23-year-old obese** female complains of **facial hair** (HIRSUTISM) that she shaves several times a week.

HPI She also complains of intermittent lower abdominal pain and heaviness off and on as well as **lack of menstruation** for the past 6 months (SECONDARY AMENORRHEA). (Patients may also show increased bleeding due to endometrial hyperplasia from unopposed estrogenic stimulation.) For the past 3 years, she has been trying to become pregnant (INFERTILITY).

PE VS: normal. PE: **obese**; increased hair on face, back, and arms; acne and frontal balding; normal breast development; no clitoromegaly; external genitalia normal; **ovaries enlarged** bilaterally; acanthosis nigricans on the axilla and neck and below the breasts.

Labs **Elevated LH**; low FSH; **increased LH-to-FSH ratio (> 3:1)**; normal prolactin; **increased free testosterone, DHEA, and androstenedione**; increased ratio of estrone to estradiol; hyperglycemia; normal or increased estrogen; decreased progesterone; progestin challenge test results in withdrawal bleeding.

Imaging US: **multiple ovarian cysts** bilaterally.

Pathogenesis Polycystic ovary disease (PCOD) is of idiopathic etiology and is associated with family history; it is also known as **Stein-Leventhal syndrome**. PCOD is characterized by **anovulatory cycles** (with loss of midcycle temperature elevation), **excess ovarian androgen** production, and multiple ovarian cysts. Obesity is common; androstenedione undergoes aromatization to estrone in fat tissue. Estrone stimulates LH and suppresses FSH secretion, which further leads to the vicious cycle of LH causing increased androgen production.

Epidemiology PCOD is the **most common cause of hirsutism** and is usually seen in females in their **late teens and young adulthood**; 30% of cases are associated with prior CNS injury and hyperprolactinemia. PCOD increases the risk of developing type 2 diabetes.

Management Rule out other possible causes of anovulation and hirsutism (e.g., thyroid disease, androgen-secreting tumors); **weight loss** results in symptomatic improvement in many patients as well as return of menses and ovulation. Estrone-positive feedback on the pituitary must be broken if the disease is to be treated correctly. **OCPs** increase steroid hormone–binding globulin and suppress the increased LH production, with a consequent decrease in free testosterone and androstenedione and the return of a regular, albeit artificial, menstruation. **Induction of ovulation** by clomiphene may be attempted. Metformin may increase ovulation as well as decrease insulin resistance.

Complications Endometrial hyperplasia and carcinoma; multiple pregnancy after clomiphene-induced ovulation.

CASE 21

ID/CC A **34-year-old** female complains of **breast pain** that is partially relieved by OTC analgesics, together with **depression**, **anxiety**, and a loss of interest in pleasurable activities (ANHEDONIA) **just prior** to **the onset of her periods**.

HPI The patient also feels "**swollen**" and **irritable** and often has **headaches** during this time. With the onset of menses these complaints disappear, but **colicky lower abdominal pain** occurs, sometimes incapacitating her (DYSMENORRHEA). She is a **smoker**, has irritable bowel syndrome, and was previously admitted for paroxysmal supraventricular tachycardia. She suffered **postpartum depression** following the birth of her two children.

PE VS: **tachycardia** (HR 110); mild hypotension (BP 100/60); mild tachypnea (RR 24); no fever. PE: well hydrated and **anxious-appearing**.

Labs CBC/UA: normal. Lytes: normal (hypoglycemia has been suggested in pathogenesis). TFTs and cortisol normal (to rule out hypo- or hyperthyroidism as well as hypopituitarism or Addison's disease).

Imaging CXR/KUB: normal. US, abdomen: no apparent pathology.

Pathogenesis Premenstrual dysphoric disorder is not fully understood and has a **multifactorial** pathogenesis involving psychiatric, physiologic, and endocrine factors such as estrogen-progesterone imbalance, hyperprolactinemia, hyperaldosteronism, and hypoglycemia. In the diagnosis of premenstrual dysphoric disorder, the **relationship of the symptoms to the menstrual period** is more important than the nature of the symptoms, since a wide constellation of symptoms are included in the disorder. Key to diagnosis is the presence of a "**disease-free period**" **during the follicular phase** of the cycle.

Epidemiology Premenstrual dysphoric disorder is seen with increasing frequency in patients with **preexisting depression** and those who suffered from **postpartum depression**. There is also a higher incidence in the fourth and fifth decades. Patients with the disorder may also have illnesses such as gastritis, colitis, migraine, asthma, allergies, and neurodermatitis.

Management The diagnosis is one of exclusion; other causes of disease must be ruled out with appropriate lab tests, psychiatric evaluation, endoscopy, and pelvic ultrasound. **Exercise**, reducing sodium intake, and pyridoxine and magnesium supplements may improve symptoms. **SSRIs** (fluoxetine), **OCPs**, **NSAIDs**, diuretics, and medroxyprogesterone may be effective if other therapies have failed. **Counseling** or referral to a mental health professional is often appropriate.

Complications Chronicity, failure of medical treatment, and periodic disability.

CASE 22

ID/CC A 20-year-old woman presents for an evaluation of **amenorrhea**.

HPI She has **never menstruated**. She complains of **swelling in the inguinal and labial region**.

PE **Tall** with **eunuchoid features; breasts large** but with sparse glandular tissue; nipples and areolae pale; **no axillary or pubic hair; bilateral inguinal hernias (ectopic testes)**; labia minora underdeveloped; vagina ends as **blind sac**.

Labs Karyotype: **46,XY**. Serum **testosterone levels normal for male**; biopsy of removed testes reveals **no evidence of spermatogenesis**.

Imaging US: **absent uterus and rudimentary fallopian tubes**; no ovaries.

Pathogenesis Testicular feminization is inherited as an **X-linked recessive trait** resulting in the **absence of testosterone receptors**; individuals have a 46,XY genotype and a female phenotype. Because müllerian inhibiting factor is secreted, these individuals have an absence of müllerian-derived structures.

Epidemiology The incidence of primary amenorrhea is < 3%, with testicular feminization accounting for 10% of all cases.

Management Patients are usually regarded socially as **female**; **gonadectomy** is performed because of the increased risk (50%) of **testicular neoplasia**. Estrogen treatment is given for maintaining secondary sexual characteristics. Surgical treatment involves creation of a vagina.

Complications Confused gender identity and infertility.

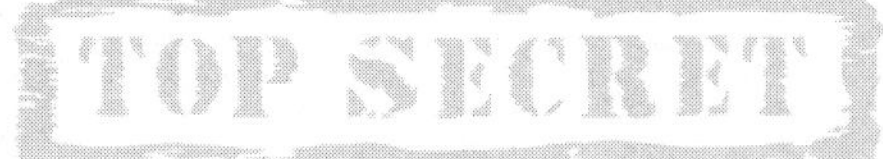

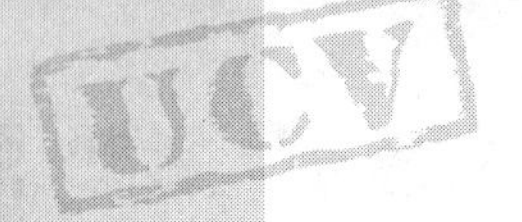

CASE 23

ID/CC A 17-year-old girl is brought by her mother to a gynecologist because her **periods have not yet begun** (PRIMARY AMENORRHEA).

HPI She underwent surgical repair for **coarctation of the aorta** a few years ago.

PE VS: normal. PE: **short in stature; low-set ears**; breasts, pubic and axillary hair, and external genitalia not developed; **short, webbed neck; shield chest** with widely spaced nipples; increased **carrying angle at elbow** (CUBITUS VALGUS).

Labs **Low estradiol; high pituitary gonadotropins** (hypergonadotropic hypergonadism). Karyotype: **45,XO** (consistent with diagnosis of Turner's syndrome).

Imaging US: **"streak" dysgenetic ovaries.**

Pathogenesis Most patients with Turner's syndrome have a **45,XO karyotype**; others have an alteration in the structure of one of the X chromosomes or exhibit a **mosaic pattern** for two or more cell lines (usually 45,X and either 46,XY or 46,XX). A mosaic pattern will result in various degrees of **gonadal dysgenesis, secondary amenorrhea, and premature menopause**; if a Y chromosome is present in the genotype, the risk of **gonadoblastomas** makes gonadectomy advisable.

Epidemiology Incidence is 1 in 2,500 live female births.

Management **Estrogen replacement therapy**. If diagnosis is made in childhood, short stature can be treated with **oxandrolone and/or growth hormone**. Cyclical use of estrogen and progesterone will initiate regular menstrual bleeding, although infertility persists.

Complications Gonadal neoplasia and infertility.

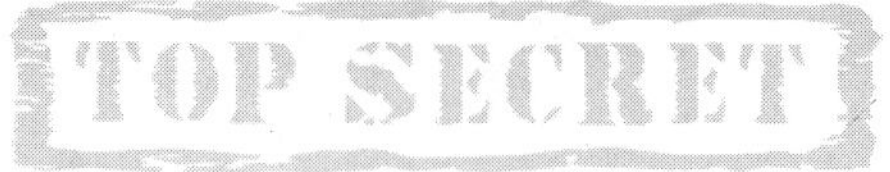

CASE 24

ID/CC A 20-year-old college student is brought to the ER after being found in an alley.

HPI The patient does not speak, and her clothes are torn and bloody.

PE VS: tachycardia (HR 110); normal BP; tachypnea (RR 20); no fever. PE: one **laceration** on scalp with dried blood; several **scratches** on face; **right eye swollen** shut and ecchymotic; lip swollen; **two front teeth missing**; chest and arms show **fingernail scratches** and several **ecchymoses and hematomas**; inner thighs reveal streaks of dried blood and semen; vulva swollen and excoriated; small branches and leaves stuck to skin of posterior legs and buttocks.

Labs CBC: normal. RPR/HIV: negative. UA: mild hematuria. Samples from throat, anus, and vagina sent for Gram stain and gonococcal and chlamydia culture; pregnancy test negative.

Imaging CXR: normal.

Pathogenesis Sexual assault constitutes an **expression of power and aggression** on the part of the perpetrator, who uses sexual acts to threaten and hurt the victim. Rape involves the **illegal penetration of any orifice in the body by hand, penis, or object**.

Epidemiology Rape is underreported; approximately half of all cases are reported. Rape may be committed by an acquaintance or spouse; **50% of rapists are known to the victim**. The vast majority of victims are women, but the number of male victims is on the rise.

Management Recognize the great **psychological trauma** of the patient. Shame, remorse, guilt, fear, and anger are initially experienced, and these are best dealt with by trained counselors. A **respectful** and **noncritical attitude** will be most beneficial to the victim. A detailed history should also be taken, including relevant obstetrical and gynecologic data such as last date of coitus (to aid in semen analysis), last menstrual period, pregnancy status, and prior STDs; a physical examination should then be completed for forensic purposes. Particulate matter should be collected as evidence (fingernail scrapings, pubic hair combings, dirt, pieces of clothing, leaves). A Wood's light will allow semen to be visualized. Obtain samples from the mouth, anus, and vagina, and record the percentage of motile sperm. Cultures for gonococcus and chlamydia should be obtained as well as a Pap smear, a *Trichomonas vaginalis* wet prep, VDRL, HIV, and pregnancy tests. **Ceftriaxone and doxycycline/azithromycin** may be given for the prevention of gonorrhea and chlamydia. Treat wounds with local care and **tetanus prophylaxis**, and **vaccinate**

continued

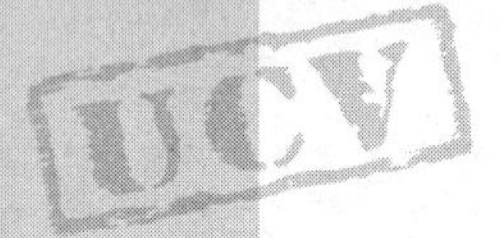

against hepatitis B. Pregnancy prophylaxis may be given with 0.5 mg of norgestrel/0.05 mg ethinylestradiol, two tabs PO in the ER and two tabs PO 12 hours afterward.

Complications

The **rape trauma syndrome** consists of immediate and chronic phases. In the immediate phase, a victim may experience severe mood swings and feelings of anger, guilt, disbelief, and denial. In the chronic phase, a victim may experience nightmares and relationship difficulties, which may be indicative of PTSD. Other complications include gonorrhea, syphilis, HIV, and pregnancy.

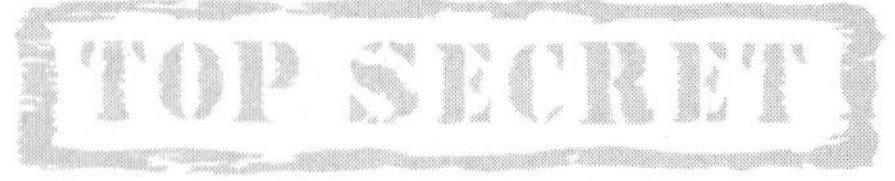

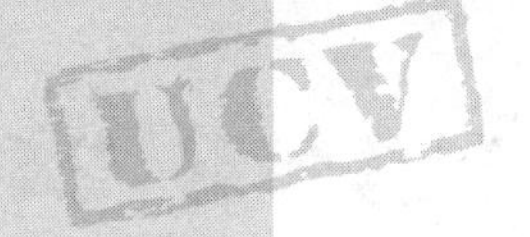

CASE 25

ID/CC A 40-year-old woman who underwent **tubal ligation 10 years ago requests reversal**; she has remarried and now wants a child.

HPI Her menstrual periods are regular, and her last delivery was 10 years ago.

PE VS: normal. PE: mini-laparotomy incision (tubal ligation); pelvic and rectal exam normal.

Labs CBC/Lytes/UA: normal. PT/PTT: normal.

Imaging CXR/KUB: normal. US, pelvis: normal uterus.

Pathogenesis Although tubal ligation is **definitive**, some patients may request reversal. Tubal ligation is performed either postpartum through a small infraumbilical incision or by laparoscopy and involves a variety of techniques, including the Pomeroy operation (performed postpartum, where a loop of tube is tied with absorbable suture, a portion is removed, and the ends separate with a gap once the suture absorbs), fimbriectomy, spring clips (HULKA CLIPS), Silastic bands (FALOPE RINGS), and electrocauterization.

Epidemiology Tubal ligation is performed twice as frequently as vasectomy. Laparoscopic tubal ligation has a failure rate of up to 1 in 100, whereas the Pomeroy operation has a failure rate of 1 in 500; all methods taken together show a failure rate of 1%. The pregnancy rate after tubal ligation decreases with time after the operation, but the ectopic pregnancy rate remains the same; 30% of the pregnancies that occur after tubal ligation are ectopic. Most failures occur in females less than 30 years of age due to fistula formation.

Management **Reanastomosis** may be tried with microsurgical techniques. Tubal reconstruction does not guarantee the return of reproductive potential and has an increased risk of **ectopic pregnancy**. **In vitro fertilization** may be an option.

Complications Bleeding, infection, and visceral injury.

TOP SECRET

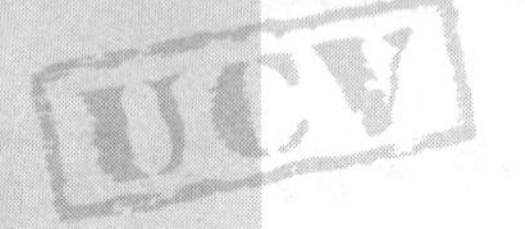

CASE 26

ID/CC A 35-year-old woman complains of **galactorrhea**, **visual field defects, and inability to conceive**.

HPI The patient has been **amenorrheic** for the past 6 months (SECONDARY AMENORRHEA) and also feels that her **field of vision** is **constricted**; she denies use of any medications or drugs. She has a healthy 7-year-old son (SECONDARY INFERTILITY), is not using any contraceptives, and wishes to conceive.

PE Visual field charting reveals **bitemporal hemianopia**; pelvic exam unremarkable; **breasts express milk** readily on pressure.

Labs Pregnancy test negative; **TSH normal**; **elevated prolactin** (> 2500 mU/L) (suggestive of macroadenoma); breast biopsy normal.

Imaging [Fig. 26A] CT: enhancing **pituitary macroadenoma** (> 10 mm) **compressing the optic chiasm.** [Fig. 26B] CT, coronal: a different case with an enhancing pituitary fossa mass.

Pathogenesis Hyperprolactinemia is defined as a prolactin level of > 800 mU/L and is considered significant when accompanied by oligomenorrhea. Hyperprolactinemia interferes with the menstrual cycle by suppressing the pulsatility of LH release from the pituitary; common causes include **prolactin-producing tumors**, **primary hypothyroidism**, **drugs** such as metoclopramide and phenothiazines, and **chronic renal failure**. It may also be **idiopathic**.

Epidemiology Prolactinomas are present in > 10% of the population.

Management **Bromocriptine** (dopamine agonist) followed by **surgical** resection; **fertility is usually restored** after treatment. For tumors < 10 mm, bromocriptine with annual CT/MR. If menses do not resume, ovulation induction may be achieved with clomiphene citrate.

Complications Infertility and panhypopituitarism.

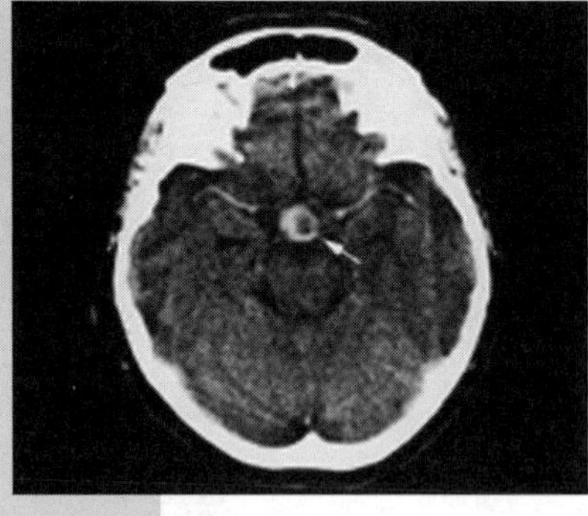

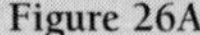

Figure 26A

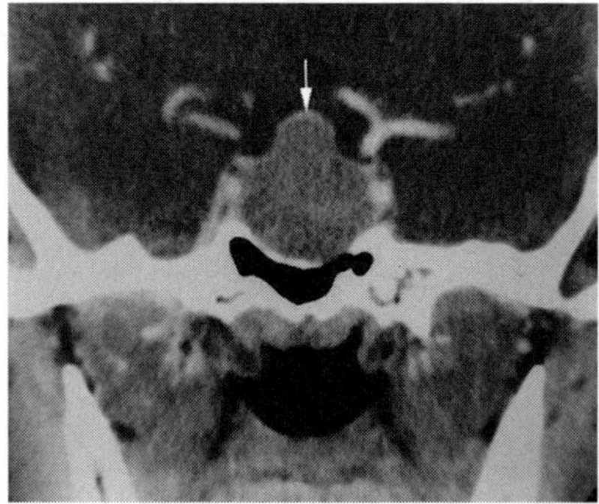

Figure 26B

CASE 27

ID/CC A 35-year-old woman presents with confusion, **abrupt-onset high fever, vomiting, diarrhea**, and **severe headache**.

HPI She developed an extensive **skin rash** 2 days ago followed by a **high-grade fever and chills** today. Her husband says she uses a **diaphragm for contraception**.

PE VS: **tachycardia** (HR 110); **fever** (39.2°C); **hypotension** (< 90 mm systolic). PE: toxic-appearing; drowsy but responding to verbal commands; **scarlatiniform rash** seen over entire body; **pharyngeal, conjunctival, and vaginal mucosae congested**; no neck rigidity or Kernig's sign; fundus normal; no localizing neurologic deficit found.

Labs CBC: **leukocytosis; anemia; thrombocytopenia** (< 100,000). UA: mild pyuria. BUN and creatinine elevated; **CPK elevated**. LFTs: **elevated bilirubin; elevated AST and ALT. Blood culture negative** (illness due to toxin, not invasion of the organism); vaginal cultures yield ***Staphylococcus aureus***. LP: CSF normal.

Pathogenesis Staphylococcal toxic shock syndrome (TSS) is the result of localized staphylococcal soft-tissue infections arising from tumors, abscesses and abrasions, burns, osteomyelitis, and postsurgical infection. The effects of the disease are mediated through the **exotoxin TSST-1**, which functions as a **superantigen**, stimulating the production of **interleukin-1** and **tumor necrosis factor** and the release of endotoxin. **Superabsorbent tampons** obstruct menstrual outflow, causing retrograde flow and peritoneal seeding with bacteria.

Epidemiology Staphylococcal TSS has been associated with the use of **vaginal contraceptive sponges and tampons. Most cases of TSS occur in menstruating women**. With the elimination of suspect superabsorbent tampons and more judicious use of ordinary tampons, the incidence of staphylococcal TSS associated with menstruation has declined; nonmenstrual causes now account for > 20% of current cases. Most patients recover in 1 to 2 weeks; the mortality rate is approximately 2%.

Management Immediate treatment of **hypotension and shock** with vigorous fluid replacement (and supplemental catecholamines if needed), drainage of any staphylococcal abscesses, and **systemic antimicrobial therapy** with a β-lactamase-resistant penicillin or a cephalosporin.

Complications Up to 30% of women may have recurrences.

CASE 28

ID/CC A 43-year-old **black** female complains of **frequent, profuse, nonpainful menstrual periods** (bleeding is the most common presenting symptom of uterine leiomyomata).

HPI The patient has been having **urinary frequency** (due to pressure on the bladder) without any pain or hematuria.

PE VS: normal. PE: no gum or subcutaneous bleeding; mild pallor; **irregular, mobile, nontender, firm pelvic mass; enlarged and irregular uterus** with multiple firm and round **nodularities** on anterior and posterior aspects; adnexa nonpalpable; no leg edema.

Labs CBC/PBS: **hypochromic, microcytic anemia** (chronic iron deficiency anemia due to increased bleeding). Normal ESR. Lytes/UA: normal. TFTs, PT/PTT, and INR: normal.

Imaging **[Fig. 28A]** US, pelvis: a large, round, hypoechoic mass is seen on the uterus. **[Fig. 28B]** US, pelvis: two discrete hypoechoic areas are seen in the uterus in another patient. **[Fig. 28C]** XR, pelvis: calcification of a fibroid is demonstrated in another patient.

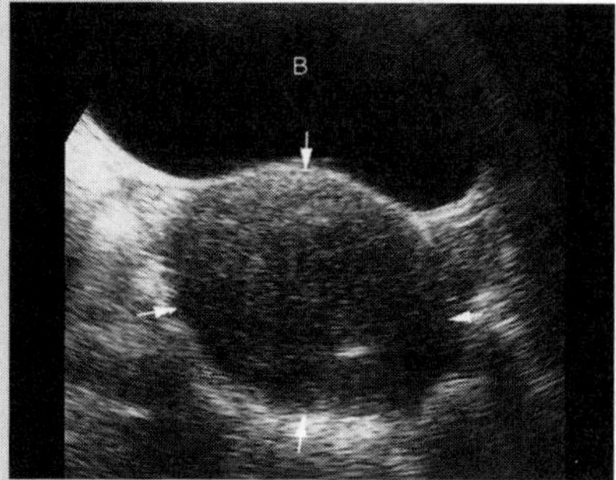

Figure 28A

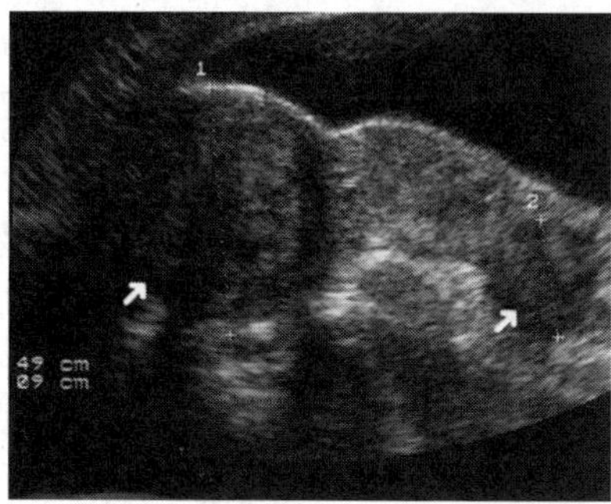

Figure 28B

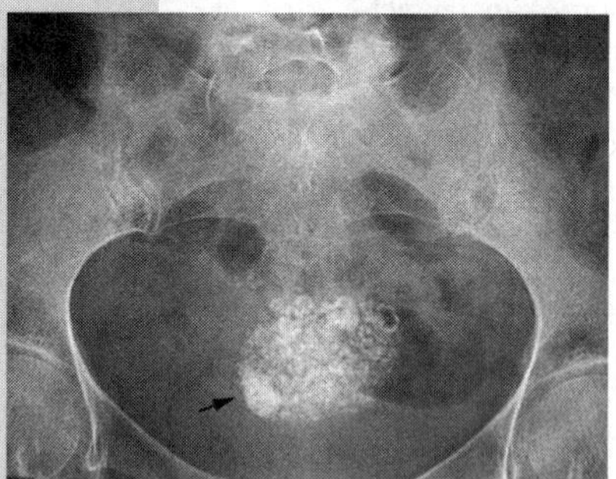

Figure 28C

continued

CASE 28

GYNECOLOGY

Pathogenesis

Leiomyomas (UTERINE FIBROIDS) are benign, **estrogen-dependent** tumors of unknown etiology consisting of myometrium. They may be **subserosal** (on the serosal side of the uterine wall), **intramural** (located in the myometrium; most common type), or **submucosal** (protruding toward the uterine cavity). Submucosal leiomyomas are most likely to cause irregular bleeding (due to distortion of the endometrium and blood supply).

Epidemiology

Fibroids are the **most common tumors affecting women** and the most common surgical indication for hysterectomy. They have a higher incidence in blacks and occur more frequently in the later premenopausal years; after menopause, they tend to atrophy and calcify.

Management

Endometrial malignancy or hyperplasia must be ruled out by **endometrial biopsy** in patients who present with bleeding during the late premenopausal or early postmenopausal period. A **Pap smear** is also indicated to rule out cervical cancer. Many cases may be managed by close observation with frequent follow-up to prevent anemia and detect tumor growth. In some patients, large leiomyomata impinging on the uterine cavity cause infertility or recurrent abortions, in which case a **myomectomy** is warranted. If a patient is symptomatic but perimenopausal, a conservative approach may be used consisting of **cyclical progestogens** or GnRH antagonists until the onset of menopause. Consider **hysterectomy** for symptomatic females who have completed childbirth. Also consider uterine artery embolization.

Complications

Complications include profuse **hemorrhage**; **pelvic pain** due to twisting of mass or infarction; **infertility**; malignant transformation (rare); hydronephrosis due to mass effect and pressure on ureters; protrusion of large submucous myomas with risk of infection; and calcific, hyaline (most common), or hemorrhagic degeneration. During pregnancy there is also an increased incidence of spontaneous abortions, preterm labor, postpartum bleeding, and breech presentations. Fibroids may undergo painful degeneration, which typically is treated by analgesics.

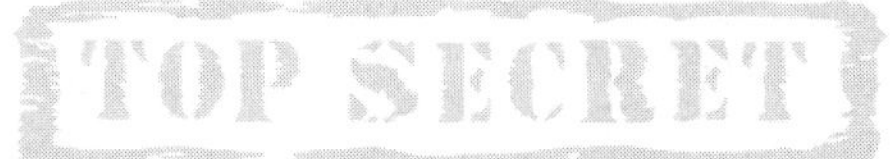

CASE 29

ID/CC A 61-year-old woman complains of a **heavy sensation** in her lower abdomen made worse by straining, increased **frequency of urination**, and **burning on urination** (DYSURIA; due to altered location of the bladder with stagnation of urine and bacterial proliferation).

HPI She is an otherwise healthy **multiparous female** whose children were all **delivered vaginally**. She has also experienced **leakage of urine while sneezing and coughing** (STRESS INCONTINENCE). She has been menopausal for 12 years and has not taken hormone replacement.

PE Inspection of external genitalia (while asking patient to bear down) reveals a mass bulging through the anterior wall of the vagina (CYSTOCELE) and downward protrusion of cervix (UTERINE PROLAPSE) (examine the patient standing so that the full extent of the protrusion can be assessed).

Labs UA: abundant leukocytes and bacteria; alkaline pH and positive nitrates (due to infection from stagnation of urine).

Imaging Voiding cystourethrogram: the bladder drops below the symphysis pubis during voiding; loss of posterior urethrovesical angle.

Pathogenesis Childbirth causes stretching of the pelvic support structures; **increased weight** during pregnancy and the **loss of muscle tone** and estrogen that accompanies menopause exacerbate incompetence of pelvic support, resulting in cystourethrocele and uterine prolapse. Aggravating factors include obesity, chronic cough, and frequent straining from constipation. If seen in nulliparity, it is usually the result of spina bifida occulta.

Epidemiology Most common in multiparous, postmenopausal women.

Management Nonsurgical treatment includes avoidance of straining and lifting heavy weights, **pessary support**, topical, oral, or parenteral **estrogens**, and **pelvic floor exercises** (KEGEL EXERCISES). **Surgery** is indicated when the patient suffers from recurrent urinary symptoms or if the cystocele is sufficiently large.

Complications Keratinization of the vagina, decubitus ulceration, cervical hypertrophy, obstructive lesions of the urinary tract, recurrent UTIs, and incarceration of the prolapse.

CASE 30

ID/CC A 30-year-old woman complains of **vaginal itching, soreness, and an odorless discharge**.

HPI The discharge is **thick, white, and curdy**. She has a history of **burning on urination** (DYSURIA). She is taking **OCPs**.

PE Thick, white discharge present on pelvic exam.

Labs Wet preparation treated with KOH reveals **presence of yeast cells and pseudohyphae**; vaginal pH normal (4.0); saline smear unremarkable. UA: negative.

Pathogenesis Factors such as **antibiotic use, pregnancy, diabetes, immunosuppression, and OCP use** can decrease the concentration of lactobacilli in the vagina, allowing for the **overgrowth of *Candida***.

Management Vaginal tablets and creams produce equal cure rates. Treat with an **imidazole** such as **miconazole** or **clotrimazole** intravaginally for 3 to 7 nights or **fluconazole orally in a single dose**. Treatment of sexual partners is not indicated.

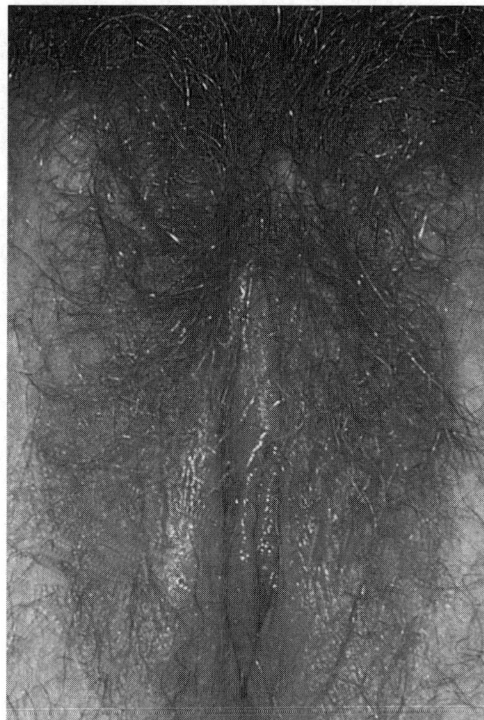

Figure 30 Inflammation of the vulva.

CASE 31

ID/CC A 35-year-old female complains of **intense vaginal itching and discomfort**.

HPI She also complains of a **malodorous, profuse, frothy greenish discharge**. She is not using any barrier contraceptives.

PE VS: normal HR and BP; no fever. PE: cervix and vaginal mucosa appear visibly irritated and inflamed; "**strawberry spots**" on vaginal wall and cervix; malodorous, frothy gray discharge confirmed.

Labs **Vaginal pH > 4.5**; saline smear reveals **presence of motile trichomonads** and PMNs (diagnostic even if only one trichomonad is seen); KOH smear unremarkable.

Pathogenesis *Trichomonas* vaginitis is caused by the **sexually transmitted *Trichomonas vaginalis***; semen, menstrual blood, or processes that alter vaginal pH increase susceptibility to infection. *Trichomonas* may also be seen on Pap smear.

Epidemiology *Trichomonas* vaginitis is as common as gonorrhea among sexually active women.

Management Treat both patient and partner with a 2-g single dose of **metronidazole**. In the first trimester of pregnancy treat with clotrimazole cream or suppository. Vinegar douching decreases parasite load and markedly reduces symptoms.

Complications Complications include cervical and vaginal epithelial changes resulting in false-positive Pap smears. Patients taking metronidazole should not drink alcohol, as it leads to a **disulfiram-like reaction**.

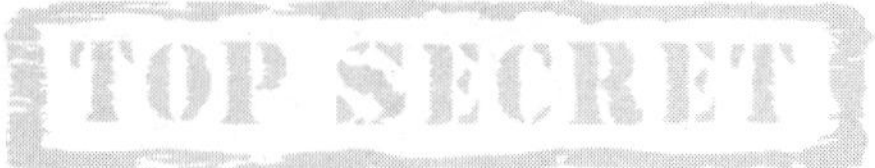

CASE 32

GYNECOLOGY

ID/CC A **63-year-old** female complains of a thick, yellowish, **purulent discharge** and a **painful lesion** on the right vulva for 2 days (carcinoma is usually painless but may be painful in the presence of secondary infection).

HPI The patient has had **vulvar pruritus** for several months, which she has been unsuccessfully treating with various creams. For the past 2 days, she has also noticed some bleeding and staining of her undergarments.

PE VS: normal. PE: no abdominal masses; inguinal area reveals **rubbery, tender nodes** on affected side (due to superimposed infection); vulva shows 2.5-cm **ulcerating lesion** on posterior aspect of right labia majora with rolled, **indurated edges**, easy bleeding, signs of local infection (erythema, increase in temperature, edema, pain), and surrounding hypopigmentation; vaginal exam reveals atrophic mucosal surface; cervix normal; no pelvic masses; rectal exam reveals normal sphincter tone with no masses.

Labs CBC: mild leukocytosis. Lytes: normal. FSH and LH elevated (due to menopause). UA: normal; urine culture and sensitivity negative. Gram stain (of exudate) reveals abundant gram-positive cocci in clusters; excisional biopsy reveals **squamous cell carcinoma**.

Imaging CXR: unfolded aortic knob; mild cardiomegaly; no infiltrates; no signs of metastatic disease. IVP: normal.

Pathogenesis Vulvar intraepithelial neoplasia (VIN) I, II, and III are considered premalignant conditions that may progress to invasive vulvar carcinoma. Risk factors include **human papillomavirus 16 and 18**, obesity, and hypertension. As in cervical cancer, VIN precedes the development of invasive carcinoma by many years. Vulvar carcinoma may be ulcerating or fungating (EXOPHYTIC) as well as macular or papular; fungating lesions or ulcers are not always seen. The most common type is **squamous cell**, which is usually well differentiated and keratinizing. Tumors invade by local extension and by lymphatic spread. The FIGO staging system is surgical, with TNM grading of the lesion as follows: **stage I**, tumor confined to the vulva/perineum (< 2 cm); **stage II**, tumor confined to the vulva/perineum (> 2 cm); **stage III**, tumor of any size with local spread (lower urethra, vagina, or anus) or unilateral lymph node involvement; **stage IV**, widespread invasion and/or bilateral lymph node involvement.

Epidemiology Comprises approximately 5% of all gynecologic malignancies and has an overall 5-year survival rate of approximately 65%. It is usually a disease of **elderly females**, with the highest incidence in the 60s.

Management Lesions of the vulva that look suspicious should be biopsied. Toluidine blue and colposcopy may help guide sites for biopsy. IVP will rule out kidney/ureteral disease and will detect possible local GU invasion;

continued

sigmoidoscopy is suggested with posterior vulvar lesions. **Vulvar intraepithelial neoplasia** may be treated by skinning vulvectomy, **wide local excision**, or laser. The verrucous type may be treated with wide local excision. For vulvar cancer, **wide radical local excision** with **bilateral inguinal lymph node dissection** is the mainstay of treatment for stages I to III. Lymph node status is the most important prognostic indicator.

Complications

Local spread with infection, bleeding; vaginal and anorectal spread; lymphatic disease (incidence of about 30%; all stages; spreads to iliac, femoral, and inguinal nodes and later to deep pelvic nodes); and recurrence after surgery.

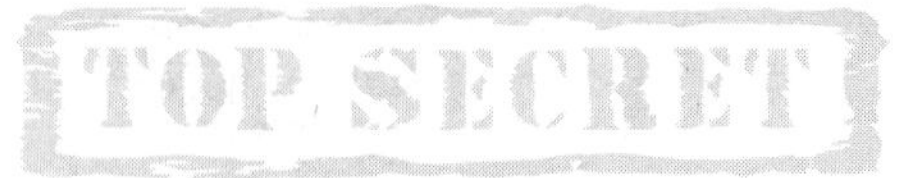

CASE 33

ID/CC A 28-year-old primigravida at **13 weeks'** gestation complains of **vaginal passage of blood clots** with **lower abdominal pain** radiating to the back.

HPI She had **vaginal spotting** 1 week ago with mild abdominal cramps. She rested for 2 days, after which her symptoms disappeared until the onset of her present complaints.

PE VS: normal. PE: no acute distress; mild **hypogastric tenderness**; abdomen soft with no rigidity; no rebound tenderness; uterus soft and increased in size with an **open cervix**.

Labs CBC/Lytes: normal. ESR: normal; pregnancy test positive. UA: few RBCs.

Imaging US: uterus increased in size; no intrauterine gestational sac.

Pathogenesis The most common causes of first-trimester spontaneous abortion are **chromosomal abnormalities** (most commonly trisomies). In the second trimester, common causes include maternal anatomic defects such as bicornuate or septate uterus, Asherman's syndrome (intrauterine synechiae after vigorous curettage), leiomyomata, incompetent cervix, placental abnormalities, drugs (cocaine, tobacco, alcohol) and toxins, and maternal illnesses such as hypo/hyperthyroidism, diabetes, SLE, and infections (toxoplasmosis, HSV, rubella, CMV).

Epidemiology Up to 50% of pregnancies are thought to end in spontaneous abortion (although only 15% to 25% are recognized); risk factors for spontaneous abortion include **multiparity**, **increasing age of mother and father**, and short span between pregnancies (< 3 months). **Threatened abortion** occurs in roughly 25% of all pregnancies.

Management All couples should receive supportive counseling regarding the pregnancy loss. Patients who have undergone abortion should be informed of **recurrence risks**. After three spontaneous abortions, **genetic counseling** is indicated. In **threatened abortion**, pelvic rest and abstinence are essential. If no fetal heart rate or gestational sac is seen on US, the fetus is evacuated. **Inevitable and incomplete abortions** are managed with D&C or vacuum suction. For **missed abortion** up to the 28th week, prostaglandin suppositories may be used to stimulate contractions. Administration of RhoGAM (Rh immune globulin) is essential to prevent isoimmunization in subsequent pregnancies if the patient's blood type is Rh negative.

Complications Retained gestational sac–placenta fragments with persistent bleeding and infection, endometritis, parametritis, septic shock, DIC, and uterine wall perforation during D&C.

CASE 34

ID/CC A **38-year-old** woman **suddenly develops laborious breathing** and lightheadedness **following a vaginal delivery**.

HPI The patient is a **multigravida** (four pregnancies) who underwent complicated delivery owing to a **large fetus**. Her falling blood pressure and tachycardia were unresponsive to fluid resuscitation.

PE VS: tachycardia (HR 110); hypotension (BP 90/60); tachypnea (RR 24). PE: **cold, clammy skin; dyspneic, cyanotic, and comatose**; weak, thready pulse; generalized tonic-clonic **convulsions** begin a few minutes afterward.

Labs CBC: **thrombocytopenia. Decreased fibrinogen; prolonged bleeding time and PT/PTT; elevated fibrin split products** (due to DIC) and D-dimers.

Imaging CXR: severe **pulmonary edema**.

Pathogenesis Amniotic fluid embolism occurs when particulate matter such as hair, fetal squama-vernix, or amniotic fluid gains access to the pulmonary circulation through lacerations in the placental membrane and rupture of uterine/placental veins, producing a pulmonary embolization. **Diagnosis is made on clinical grounds**, since the presence of squamous cells in maternal blood is not enough to confirm a diagnosis of amniotic fluid embolism. Embolization produces severe, acute **pulmonary hypertension with hypoxemia**. The second phase gives rise to **acute heart failure and DIC a few hours afterward**.

Epidemiology Amniotic fluid embolism is a rare complication occurring in 1 per 50,000 deliveries (after vaginal delivery, abortion, or C-section). If it occurs in the delivery period, it may be associated with **abruptio placentae** and fetal death. Predisposing factors include **older age**, uterine rupture, and twin pregnancy with uterine overdistention.

Management Admission to the ICU, hemodynamic monitoring, oxygen, ventilatory support, treatment of acute heart failure, treatment of DIC.

Complications Death in 80% of cases; neurologic damage due to hypoxia in survivors.

CASE 35

OBSTETRICS

ID/CC A 31-year-old woman complains of **easy fatigability** and **lack of stamina for daily activities**; she has also had an unusual **urge to eat ice** (PAGOPHAGIA) **and clay** (PICA).

HPI She is a 20-week primigravida with an unremarkable medical history.

PE VS: mild tachycardia (HR 105). PE: **pallor** of mucous membranes; fetal heart rate normal (140/min).

Labs CBC: **microcytic, hypochromic** (MCHC < 30) anemia (may be normochromic or normocytic with concomitant folate deficiency); low hematocrit. [**Fig. 35**] PBS: hypochromic and microcytic RBCs; poikilocytosis. **Low serum iron level; low transferrin saturation index** (< 16%); **increased TIBC; low ferritin level**. UA/Lytes: normal. Glucose normal.

Imaging US, abdomen: 20-week intrauterine pregnancy.

Pathogenesis Iron deficiency anemia is anemia (Hct < 30% or Hb < 10 gm/dL) caused by lack of iron, resulting from diminished consumption, decreased absorption, increased demand (short interval between pregnancies), blood loss (hemorrhage), or a combination thereof. In pregnancy, iron absorption is usually increased (as opposed to folate) to offset increased demand. Because ferritin is the storage form of iron, **ferritin level is the test of choice in the diagnosis of iron deficiency** anemia.

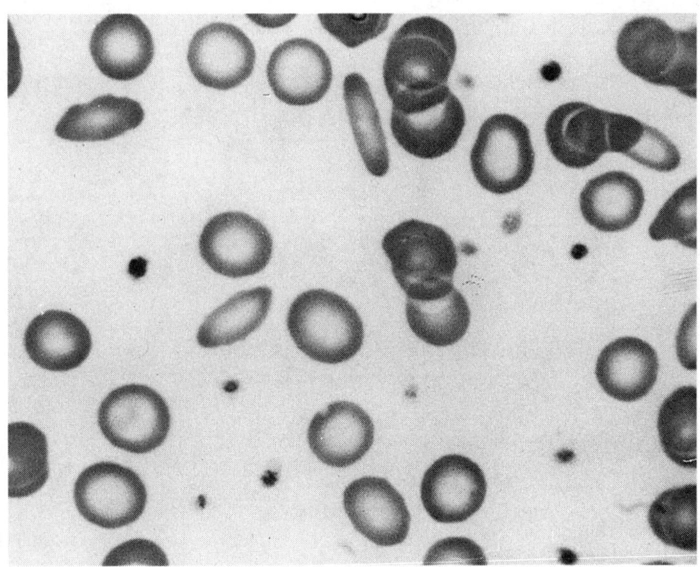

Figure 35

continued

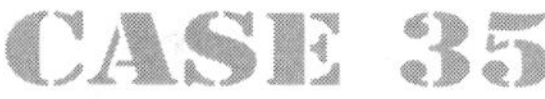

Epidemiology One-fifth of all pregnancies are associated with some degree of anemia, and iron deficiency is the most common cause of anemia in pregnancy (75%).

Management Most pregnant patients receive daily supplemental iron in prenatal vitamin preparations, and this usually suffices for prophylaxis of overt anemia. If iron deficiency anemia is established, 325 mg of ferrous sulfate should be given three times a day. Administration of iron together with vitamin C increases absorption; taking it with antacids, calcium, or meals decreases absorption. Iron-dextran may be given IM if a patient cannot tolerate iron PO.

Complications PO iron supplementation may cause black stools, epigastric discomfort, and constipation (often given with stool softeners). IM iron-dextran administration may cause local pain or anaphylaxis.

CASE 36

ID/CC A 28-year-old in her first trimester, routine office visit.

HPI This is the patient's second pregnancy; the first resulted in a normal full-term vaginal delivery.

PE VS: normal. PE: **pallor**; ejection murmur 1/6 in aortic area; pregnant uterus **with two fetuses**, each with normal fetal heart rate; no leg edema; normal neurologic and pelvic exams.

Labs CBC/PBS: **low hemoglobin** with **increased MCV** (MEGALOBLASTIC ANEMIA); leukopenia; thrombocytopenia; **hypersegmented neutrophils. Decreased reticulocyte count**; decreased serum and erythrocyte folate levels. Normocytic, normochromic anemia is also common as a result of the dilutional effects of intravascular volume expansion (PHYSIOLOGIC ANEMIA OF PREGNANCY).

Imaging US: normal development of one fetus with a slight decrease in somatometry of the second; normal amniotic fluid and placenta; no other apparent abnormalities.

Pathogenesis In pregnancy, folate demands increase fourfold and folate absorption is decreased. **Phenytoin** and **phenobarbital** therapy, spherocytosis, hemoglobinopathies with **hemolysis, multiple gestation**, and a lack of fresh green vegetables are all predisposing factors for **megaloblastic anemia of pregnancy due to folate deficiency**. Iron deficiency is also commonly present, and a normocytic anemia may appear. The best lab test to establish the diagnosis is **RBC folate level**.

Epidemiology The **most common cause of megaloblastic anemia in pregnancy** is **folate deficiency**, which constitutes about 10% of cases of pregnancy-related anemias. It usually appears in the third trimester.

Management Folate deficiency in pregnancy may be prevented with 1 mg of folic acid per day, which is also the **best preventive measure against** the development of **neural tube defects** (recommended two months prior to conception). **Reticulocytosis** is an early sign of adequate folate replacement (also give iron if the reticulocyte count does not increase after 1 week). For high-risk pregnancies (e.g., prior birth with neural tube defects or anticonvulsant drugs), give 4 **mg/day** beginning 3 months prior to pregnancy.

Complications Neural tube defects, placental abruption, and spontaneous abortion.

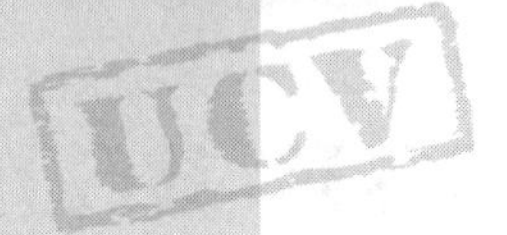

CASE 37

ID/CC A 25-year-old primigravida in her early **third trimester** complains of excessive **pruritus** and **jaundice**.

HPI The patient has been passing **dark urine** (with light-colored stool) and has no history of prior jaundice, biliary colic, or dyspepsia. She is not taking any drugs and has no history of hematemesis, melena, hematochezia, or altered sensorium. She has had an uncomplicated pregnancy up to this time.

PE VS: tachycardia (HR 105); normal BP; no fever. PE: **icterus; scratch marks** on skin; fundal height at **28 cm**; fetal parts palpable; fetal heart heard.

Labs LFTs: **elevated serum bilirubin, predominantly conjugated; elevated alkaline phosphatase** to > 10 times normal value; **AST** and **ALT** moderately **elevated**. Serologic markers for viral hepatitis A, B, and C negative; liver biopsy reveals **intrahepatic cholestasis**.

Imaging US, abdomen: no evidence of cholelithiasis or choledocholithiasis; single live fetus seen.

Pathogenesis Intrahepatic cholestasis is a hereditary metabolic defect of the liver that is usually seen in the third trimester of pregnancy; it is aggravated by high estrogen levels and is associated with OCP use. These changes resolve following delivery but recur in subsequent pregnancies.

Management Ursodeoxycholic acid inhibits the absorption of bile salts and increases their biliary secretion. Pruritus (due to elevated serum bile salts) can be treated with cholestyramine or antihistamines. **Close prenatal and intrapartum** monitoring is necessary, and early delivery may be considered once fetal maturity is established.

Complications **Significant fetal morbidity** may result, including stillbirth, premature birth, intrapartum fetal distress, and meconium-stained amniotic fluid.

TOP SECRET

CASE 38

ID/CC A 33-year-old woman in her **36th week of pregnancy** complains of new-onset **abdominal pain with fever and chills**.

HPI She is a **smoker** with no medical history. She reports that "**some water**" **ran down her thighs 24 hours ago** (smoking increases incidence of premature rupture of membranes, or PROM).

PE VS: **fever** (39.5°C); **tachycardia** (HR 110); normal BP. PE: in acute distress; **uterine tenderness**; thick, yellowish-green **cervical discharge**; cervical dilatation 3 cm; **fluid nitrazine paper test positive** (amniotic fluid, alkaline pH); **positive ferning** (sodium chloride in amniotic fluid crystallizes); **fetal tachycardia** (HR 160) with loss of variability and no decelerations.

Labs CBC: anemia; leukocytosis (16,000) with neutrophilia. UA/Lytes: normal. TFTs: normal.

Imaging US: **scant amniotic fluid** (due to PROM); no fetal abnormalities except for tachycardia.

Pathogenesis Chorioamnionitis, or **infection of the fetal membrane**, is most frequently caused by ascending infections and hematogenous spread. The most common causative organisms are **group B streptococcus, anaerobic streptococci, *Escherichia coli*, and *Bacteroides***. Risk factors include nulliparity, PROM, prolonged labor, preexisting infections, and multiple digital vaginal examinations.

Epidemiology Chorioamnionitis complicates about 1% of all deliveries. In PROM of >18 hours, there is a significantly higher incidence of chorioamnionitis; in preterm PROM the incidence may reach 25%.

Management **Antibiotic therapy** includes ampicillin, gentamicin, and clindamycin. Antibiotics are adjusted according to culture results. Delivery (induction or C-section) may be indicated based on fetal lung maturity.

Complications Failure to progress, C-section, endometritis (signs of infection that persist longer than 24 hours after delivery), myometritis, parametritis, septicemia, DIC, renal shutdown, and ARDS.

TOP SECRET

CASE 39

ID/CC A 35-year-old pregnant woman is admitted because of a **complicated obstetric history with gestational diabetes**.

HPI The patient is at 10 weeks' gestation. **During her first pregnancy she had gestational diabetes** and was prescribed insulin; her first pregnancy resulted in sudden unexpected fetal death at 36 weeks. Her second pregnancy resulted in a term **macrosomic infant weighing 4,500 g following a difficult vaginal delivery**; the baby suffered intraventricular hemorrhage and died shortly after birth. During both pregnancies, the patient had **irregular prenatal care** and **did not adhere to her insulin schedule**. Her **father is diabetic**.

PE VS: normal. PE: **obese**; pelvic exam reveals 10-week uterus; fetal heart heard on doppler.

Labs Fasting blood **glucose 160 mg/dL** (if value is < 140 mg/dL, retest at 24 to 28 weeks; if value is > 140 mg/dL, proceed to glucose tolerance test). UA: **glucosuria. Glucose tolerance test is consistent with gestational diabetes**. (In the 3-hour glucose tolerance test, 100 g of glucose is administered orally and serial blood glucose levels are checked at fasting, 1-, 2-, and 3-hour intervals. The following are considered **abnormally high values: fasting > 95 mg/dL; 1 hr > 180 mg/dL; 2 hr > 155 mg/dL; 3 hr > 140 mg/dL**. If the patient has abnormal glucose levels at any two of these four time points, gestational diabetes is diagnosed.)

Imaging US, pelvis: single, intrauterine fetus at 10 weeks with evidence of fetal heart activity.

Pathogenesis Gestational diabetes is caused by insulin resistance during pregnancy that is thought to be due to human placental lactogen (which blocks insulin receptors) and elevated circulating estrogen and progesterone.

Epidemiology Gestational diabetes must be suspected in all women with a prior history of gestational diabetes; with **significant glucosuria** on two occasions prenatally or in a single fasting urine sample; with a family history of diabetes; with previous babies weighing > 90th percentile for gestational age and sex; or with a history of previous unexpected perinatal death, polyhydramnios, or maternal obesity. **Routine prenatal screening** (serum glucose one hour following 50 g oral glucose) **is recommended at 24 to 28 weeks for all women and at initial visit for women who are at increased risk** (see predisposing factors above). Women with gestational diabetes are at increased risk of developing diabetes in the future and should be screened for diabetes 6 weeks postpartum.

continued

CASE 39

Management Prescribe the ADA diet; institute **insulin therapy with strict blood glucose monitoring** when necessary. Oral hypoglycemics are contraindicated during pregnancy because they cross the placenta and produce fetal hypoglycemia. Perform regular prenatal checkups and tests (including glucose profiles, urinalysis, and glycosylated hemoglobin), and use US to screen the fetus for malformations.

Complications **Maternal risks** include **retinopathy**, **nephropathy**, **neuropathy**, and increased risk of **polyhydramnios**, **preeclampsia**, and **UTIs**. **Fetal risks** include **congenital malformations** (cardiac and craniospinal defects); **sacral agenesis** (a rare anomaly specifically associated with diabetes); **sudden unexpected fetal death** during the last 4 to 6 weeks of pregnancy; difficult delivery (shoulder dystocia) due to **macrosomia**; and neonatal problems such as **birth trauma**, **hyaline membrane disease**, **hypoglycemia**, hypomagnesemia, **hypocalcemia**, and **jaundice**. All risks are increased by poor glycemic control, especially if ketoacidosis develops.

CASE 40

ID/CC A 20-year-old woman complains of **nausea**, especially in the morning, and **fatigue**.

HPI Her **last menstrual period was 10 weeks ago**, and she had repeated unprotected intercourse approximately 3 months ago. Her menstrual periods have previously been regular with average flow and no dysmenorrhea. She has also noted **increased frequency of micturition** (due to an increase in GFR).

PE VS: normal. PE: **breasts full and tender**; pelvic exam reveals a **soft cervix** (GOODELL'S SIGN) that is **congested and cyanotic** (CHADWICK'S SIGN); on bimanual examination, cervix and uterine body feel like two separate organs (due to **marked softening of the isthmus**) (HEGAR'S SIGN); uterus enlarged to 10 to 12 weeks' size.

Labs **Urine pregnancy test (hCG agglutination inhibition) positive**. (Quantitative hCG assays in maternal blood are extremely sensitive and may confirm pregnancy in patients where the diagnosis is uncertain.)

Imaging **[Fig. 40A]** US, pelvis: a different case in which a 6-week gestation is demonstrated. **[Fig. 40B]** US, abdomen: a gestation of 16 weeks is shown in another patient; note the abdomen (1) and head (2).

Management Inform the patient of the pregnancy and give appropriate advice regarding **drugs** (to prevent teratogenic insult), **nutrition** (a balanced diet and supplementation with iron and folic acid), **exercise** (moderate exercise along with avoidance of strenuous work), **travel** (avoidance of long-distance travel before 12 weeks and after 28 weeks), and **regular prenatal care** (monthly intervals until 32 weeks, then every 2 weeks until 36 weeks, and every week thereafter). At the initial prenatal visit, the following labs should be ordered: CBC; blood grouping and cross-matching; rubella antibody titer; cervical gonorrhea and chlamydia cultures; VDRL;

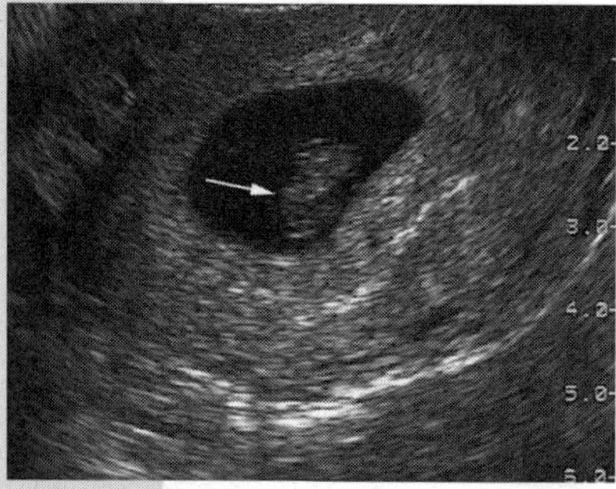

Figure 40A

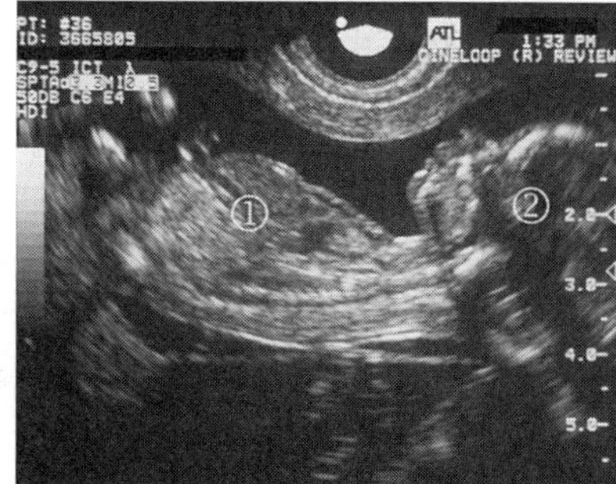

Figure 40B

continued

CASE 40

HBsAg; Pap smear; UA for glucose, protein, and microscopic exam; PPD; blood glucose; and ELISA for HIV. Standard procedures that are routinely performed after the initial visit include the following. **Before 12 weeks**: transvaginal ultrasound is the most accurate means of estimating gestational age (intrauterine gestational sac with a fetal pole and positive heartbeat can be identified as early as 6 weeks of gestation). At **15 to 20 weeks**: triple screen as follows: (1) maternal serum α-fetoprotein (AFP); (2) hCG; and (3) unconjugated estriol to identify neural tube defects (elevated AFP, low hCG, and elevated estriol), trisomy 21 (low AFP, elevated hCG, and low estriol), or trisomy 18 (low AFP, low hCG, and low estriol). At **18 to 20 weeks**: US to assess fetal development. At **24 to 28 weeks**: glucose tolerance test (one at initial visit if risk factors are present). At **28 to 30 weeks**: RhoGAM administered to Rh-negative patients. At **34 to 38 weeks**: CBC repeated. At **36 to 40 weeks**: cervical chlamydia, gonorrhea, and VDRL (in high-risk patients) and group B streptococcus cultures (in all patients).

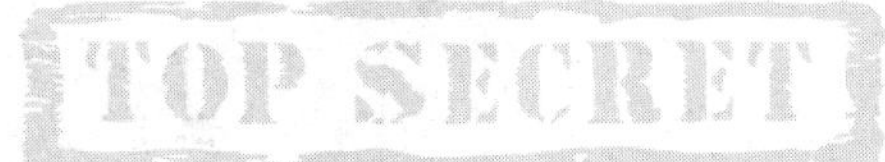

CASE 41

ID/CC A 32-year-old female presents with vaginal bleeding, **lightheadedness**, nausea, vomiting, and **fainting** after **sudden-onset left lower quadrant abdominal pain** 2 hours ago; the pain radiates to the scapular region and to the back (diaphragmatic irritation due to tubal rupture).

HPI Several years ago, the patient was using an **IUD**. She has a history of **recurrent cervicitis and PID** due to *Neisseria gonorrhoeae* and had an appendectomy during childhood. Her **last menstrual period was 39 days ago**, but she states that she is regular and never misses a period.

PE VS: **tachycardia** (HR 110); **orthostatic hypotension (BP 100/60 seated, 80/40 standing)**; tachypnea (RR 24); low-grade fever. PE: marked **pallor**; **delayed capillary refill**; abdomen distended; **tender left iliac fossa** with voluntary guarding and **rebound tenderness; decreased bowel sounds**; pelvic exam reveals mild **tenderness on cervical motion** and soft, **tender left adnexal mass**; culdocentesis reveals **nonclotting blood in cul-de-sac** (**transvaginal ultrasound** is replacing culdocentesis **for diagnosis** of ectopic pregnancy).

Labs CBC: mild anemia (due to intraperitoneal bleeding); leukocytosis. Lytes: normal. Increased BUN. UA: normal. Urine and serum pregnancy test positive. Quantitative serial serum **β-hCG** shows prolonged doubling time, plateauing or decreasing levels (as compared with a normal pregnancy); blood type O negative.

Imaging **[Fig. 41]** US, transvaginal: the ectopic gestation sac (1) is seen to be outside the empty uterus (2).

Pathogenesis Ectopic pregnancy is implantation of the fertilized ovum outside the uterine cavity, usually in the ampullary region of the fallopian tubes, followed in frequency of occurrence by the isthmus, fimbria, and interstitial portion (part of the tube that traverses the uterine wall). Ova may also implant in the cervix, the abdominal cavity, and the ovaries. The classic

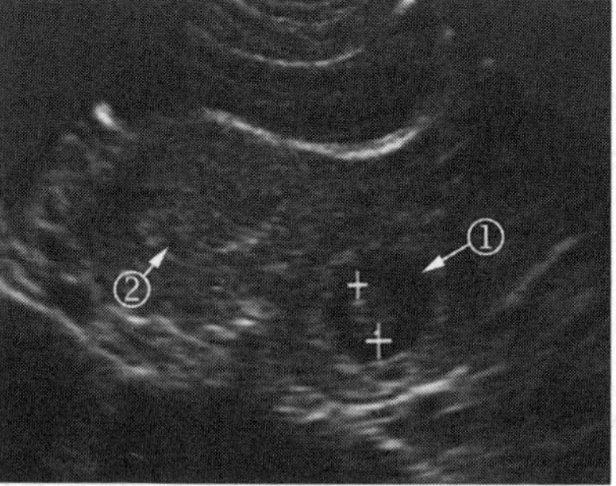

Figure 41

continued

triad in ectopic pregnancy consists of **lower abdominal pain, amenorrhea, and vaginal bleeding**, but this triad is not always found. Interstitial pregnancy ruptures later, with more profuse bleeding than other tubal pregnancies.

Epidemiology Ectopic pregnancies have increased in incidence concomitantly with PID and are the **second leading cause of maternal mortality**. Hispanics and blacks have an increased incidence of ectopic pregnancy. Risk factors include **tubal ligation**, **PID** with scarring, **IUD** use, previous ectopic pregnancy, previous complicated appendicitis with peritonitis, endometriosis, multiparity, perimenopausal years, exposure to DES, and induction of ovulation.

Management After hemodynamic stabilization (blood transfusion, etc.), a laparoscopy will confirm the diagnosis. An attempt at conservative surgery may be made laparoscopically by **salpingostomy** with removal of the product of conception or by **salpingectomy**. If the mother is Rh negative, then administer RhoGAM to prevent Rh isoimmunization. In the event of an unruptured ectopic pregnancy of < 3.5 cm, **methotrexate** may be given to induce abortion.

Complications Risk of maternal exsanguination and death; increased incidence of future ectopic pregnancies and infertility due to tubal scarring.

CASE 42

ID/CC

A 27-year-old **primigravida** complains of persistent, severe vomiting and **excessive morning nausea and vomiting** of 1 month's duration.

HPI

Five weeks ago she tested positive on a urine pregnancy test. She has been amenorrheic for 12 weeks, and her **food and water intake has been markedly reduced** owing to persistent nausea. She shows evidence of **weight loss** of about 7 pounds over the past month.

PE

VS: **tachycardia** (HR 105); **orthostatic hypotension**. PE: appears ill and moderately **dehydrated**; abdominal exam reveals fundal height to be at level of pelvic brim (12 weeks); fetal heart heard via doppler.

Labs

Serum hCG elevated (commensurate with period of gestation). Lytes: hyponatremia; hypokalemia. Abnormal TFTs (up to 60% of women with severe hyperemesis gravidarum have a transient elevation of T_4). ABGs: **hypochloremic metabolic alkalosis**. UA: positive **ketones**. Further blood tests confirm **ketonemia**.

Imaging

US, pelvis: single, live intrauterine 12-week gestation with positive fetal heart activity.

Pathogenesis

The cause of vomiting is thought to be high estrogen and β-hCG levels. Hyperemesis gravidarum is diagnosed when protracted vomiting is associated with dehydration and ketonuria.

Epidemiology

Seventy percent of all women, mostly primigravidae, complain of nausea and vomiting during early pregnancy. Hyperemesis gravidarum occurs in 4 out of 1,000 patients and tends to recur.

Management

Hospitalize and make NPO for 48 hours. Administer IV fluids (preferably glucose-saline); maintain electrolyte balance; if necessary, give antiemetics (prochlorperazine, promethazine). After correction of acidosis, start gradual oral feeding and treat nausea with pyridoxine. Other causes of hyperemesis must be ruled out.

Complications

In advanced cases, **renal and hepatic function may be compromised** (known as the toxemic phase of vomiting); in such cases and in cases that are resistant to intensive antiemetic therapy, **termination of pregnancy may be required**.

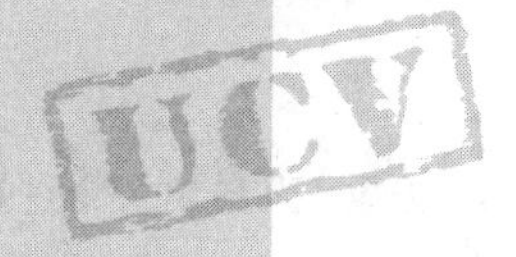

CASE 43

ID/CC A **40-year-old multipara** at 36 weeks' gestation complains of **considerable vaginal bleeding.**

HPI The bleeding is **bright red** but **painless** and of **sudden onset at rest**. The patient did not feel any uterine contractions, and the bleeding ceased after about an hour. For the past 28 weeks she has had **recurrent episodes of small amounts of vaginal bleeding**; these episodes were not preceded by trauma or intercourse, were painless, and stopped on their own. She is G7P6; the first four pregnancies were delivered vaginally and the last **two by cesarean section** (due to fetal distress and malpresentation).

PE VS: normal. PE: **no tenderness** on abdominal exam; **uterus relaxed**; no contractions felt; **vaginal exam not performed** owing to risk of provoking bleeding.

Labs CBC: normal. Blood grouped and cross-matched; **coagulation profile normal**; amniocentesis performed to **confirm fetal lung maturity** (lecithin-to-sphingomyelin ratio > 2:1).

Imaging US, abdomen: **total placenta previa** (placenta covering the cervical os) and a single live fetus in breech presentation and longitudinal lie; the biophysical profile (measure of fetal tone, movements, respiration, amniotic fluid index, fetal heart accelerations) is suggestive of fetal well-being.

Pathogenesis No definite etiology is known. With US, placenta previa can be diagnosed early in pregnancy. **Asymptomatic placenta previa or low-lying placenta detected in the second trimester should be followed closely. Many migrate upward** and resolve as the uterus enlarges, while others remain in place; bleeding in a true placenta previa is physiologic and inevitable once the cervix begins to efface.

Epidemiology Placenta previa occurs in about 0.5% of pregnancies; **predisposing factors** include **age > 35 years, multiparity, previous multiple abortions, previous cesarean sections, upper uterine cavity abnormalities, multiple gestation**, and **smoking**.

Management Hospitalization; rule out local lesions of cervix and vagina; rule out abruptio placentae and refrain from sexual intercourse. Indications for an emergent cesarean section in cases of placenta previa include persistent labor, bleeding > 500 mL, unstable bleeding requiring multiple transfusions, coagulation defects, documented fetal lung maturity, and a 36-week period of gestation. Before 36 weeks of gestation, steroids may be used to accelerate fetal lung maturity.

Complications **Maternal complications** include hemorrhage, shock, death, or placenta accreta (abnormal implantation of chorionic villi into the myometrium; risk increases with previous cesarean section). **Fetal complications** include prematurity, blood loss, and death due to asphyxia or birth injury.

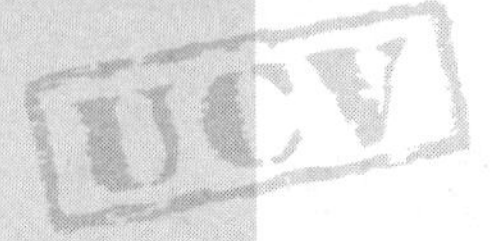

CASE 44

ID/CC A 30-year-old primigravida is brought to the emergency room with **continuous, painful vaginal bleeding**.

HPI On admission, she began to **bleed from the IV site and from the nose**. She is calculated to be at 35 weeks' gestation and admits to **smoking** and **abusing cocaine**; she has also been **hypertensive** (cocaine induced) for the past month. She has had no prior episodes of similar vaginal bleeding but has a history of **physical abuse** by her husband.

PE VS: **hypotension** (BP 100/60); **tachycardia** (HR 105). PE: looks extremely ill; epistaxis noted; abdominal exam reveals **tense uterus with marked tenderness; fetal heart audible but bradycardic** (HR 115); heavily blood-stained sanitary pad in place.

Labs CBC/PBS: **thrombocytopenia**; fragmented RBCs. Coagulation profile reveals **prolonged clot retraction time, elevated fibrinogen degradation products, hypofibrinogenemia, prolonged PT/PTT and thrombin time**, and decreased anti-thrombin III and plasminogen.

Imaging US, abdomen: significant **placental abruption with a large retroplacental clot**.

Pathogenesis Placental abruption is caused by premature separation of a normally implanted placenta before the third stage of labor. With intramyometrial infiltration of blood, the entire uterus appears matted and purplish (COUVELAIRE UTERUS) and may lead to postpartum hemorrhage.

Epidemiology The incidence of placental abruption is 1%; it is classified into marginal, partial, or total abruption and is the second most common cause of third-trimester bleeding. **Predisposing factors** include **preeclampsia, history of previous abruption, chronic hypertension, advanced maternal age, smoking and cocaine abuse, trauma**, and **sudden decrease in uterine volume** (such as that caused by ruptured membranes in polyhydramnios and after delivery of the first twin).

Management **Fluid, blood, and cryoprecipitate** (for replacement of fibrinogen if bleeding complications occur) replacement; **immediate delivery** by cesarean section is indicated in cases of severe bleeding or fetal distress. Control coagulation defects to limit bleeding during the postpartum period.

Complications **Hemorrhagic shock** (sometimes due to concealed hemorrhage into a large retroplacental clot), **coagulopathy** (DIC occurs in 3% of severe abruptions), **ischemic necrosis of distant organs** (ATN, Sheehan's syndrome), **postpartum hemorrhage, increased risk of recurrence in subsequent pregnancies, fetal anemia**, and fetal death.

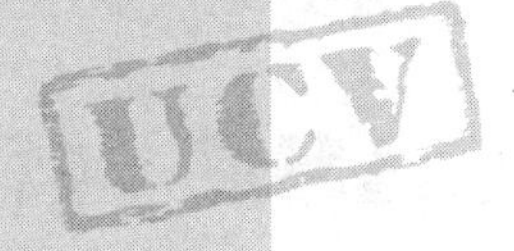

CASE 45

ID/CC A 28-year-old woman presents to a family clinic with **weight gain** and **difficulty breathing**.

HPI Her last menstrual period was 24 weeks ago. She had a normal full-term pregnancy and delivered a healthy male baby vaginally 3 years ago; she has no history of any abortions or stillbirths. She has no history of diabetes or hypertension, and her blood group is B positive. Her current pregnancy was diagnosed at home via urine testing, and she sought no prenatal care.

OBSTETRICS

PE VS: tachycardia (HR 105); normal BP; tachypnea (RR 24). PE: no pallor, icterus, or pedal edema; abdominal exam reveals markedly distended abdomen; **fundal height corresponds to 32 weeks**' gestation (calculated at 24 weeks); **fluid thrill** palpable in all directions; **distant and feeble fetal heart sounds** audible.

Labs **Serum α-fetoprotein (AFP)** (ideally should have been done at 15 to 20 weeks of gestation) **elevated; screening test for gestational diabetes negative** (polyhydramnios is frequently associated with maternal diabetes).

Imaging US, abdomen: polyhydramnios (**amniotic fluid index greater than 20**) and **anencephalic fetus**.

Pathogenesis Polyhydramnios is diagnosed on the basis of **an amniotic fluid index of more than 25**. Although its exact cause is not known, it is strongly associated with **uniovular twin pregnancy**, in which the hydramnios affects only one amniotic sac (usually the upper); **neural tube defects** such as **anencephaly** and **spina bifida**; congenital esophageal defects such as tracheoesophageal fistula, duodenal atresia, or pyloric stenosis; **maternal diabetes** and **cardiac** or **renal disease**; hydrops fetalis; and **chorioangioma of the placenta**, a rare tumor that generally presents with an acute polyhydramnios. **Polyhydramnios is invariably present when there is an open defect allowing free communication with the CSF**.

Epidemiology Affects 1% of all pregnancies. Neural tube defects vary from anencephaly, encephalocele, and meningomyelocele to spina bifida.

Management Frequent US examinations; perform therapeutic amniocentesis in the presence of maternal respiratory compromise/marked uterine distention. Tocolysis if premature labor ensues; deliver if fetus is mature. To detect neural tube defects, **maternal serum AFP is recommended as a routine screening prenatal test at 15 to 20 weeks of pregnancy**; an elevated level of maternal serum AFP is followed, with amniotic fluid AFP, acetylcholinesterase levels, and an obstetric US to confirm the diagnosis. **Folic acid supplementation** is recommended for the next pregnancy to reduce the risk of neural tube defects.

Complications Preterm labor, maternal respiratory distress, umbilical cord prolapse, abruptio placentae, and fetal malpresentation.

CASE 46

ID/CC A 30-year-old woman complains of **cessation of menses** (AMENORRHEA) for 2 months along with a feeling of **fullness in her breasts, early-morning nausea, and vomiting** (PREGNANCY).

HPI The patient is the mother of a child who was born of a normal vaginal delivery 3 years ago; 4 months ago she had an **IUD** (Progestasert) inserted.

PE VS: normal. PE: **IUD in place** with **strings visible** on speculum exam.

Labs CBC/Lytes: normal. **Pregnancy test positive**. UA: normal; urine culture and sensitivity normal.

Imaging US, pelvis: IUD inside uterus; product of conception implanted on the uterine fundus.

Pathogenesis The IUD is one of the most effective methods of reversible contraception (failure rate is < 2% per 6 years of use). IUDs prevent the implantation of the fertilized ovum by creating a hostile endometrium (subclinical endometritis) via an inflammatory response to the foreign body; they also exert a spermicidal action through increased phagocytosis. IUDs may contain copper (spermicidal) or progesterone (direct action on the endometrium; needs to be changed annually) for added effectiveness. Ideally, they are inserted during menstruation. **Advantages** are the ability to confer **long-term (up to 10 years) contraception** with only periodic checkups and obviating the need for patient compliance with medications. **Contraindications** include pregnancy, previous septic abortion (within 3 months), gynecologic infections, multiple sexual partners, abnormal Pap smears, uterine malformations, and Wilson's disease (with copper-containing IUDs).

Epidemiology Of the rare pregnancies that occur with IUDs, 1 in 20 is septic. The rate of spontaneous abortion may be increased up to 40% for women with an IUD in place. Given this, the device needs to be removed if continuation of pregnancy is desired. IUDs are not associated with an increased risk of congenital malformations. After an IUD has been removed, 90% of patients not using other forms of contraception become pregnant within a year.

Management If the patient wants to continue the pregnancy and strings are visible, the IUD must be gently removed. If the strings are not visible and no part of the IUD is located near the cervical os for easy grasping, the device may be left in place with careful periodic observation. The incidence of spontaneous abortion with an IUD in place is 50%.

continued

CASE 46

Complications Risks of IUD usage include perforation of the uterine fundus during insertion (1:2,000), spontaneous expulsion (10%; highest incidence during the first year after placement), increased menstrual flow and intermenstrual bleeding, dysmenorrhea (sometimes incapacitating), pregnancy, ectopic pregnancy (5% of IUD-related pregnancies), and increased incidence of PID (with multiple sexual partners).

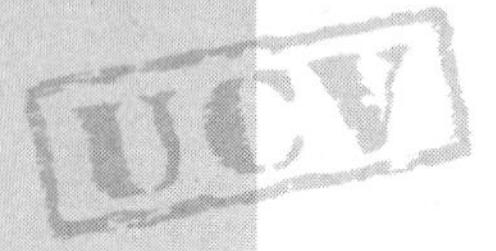

CASE 47

ID/CC A 30-year-old woman presents with **fever**, malaise, and **lower abdominal pain** 5 days **following a cesarean section**.

HPI Her **lochia (uterine discharge) has become purulent** and is particularly **foul-smelling**. She does not complain of breast discomfort, dysuria, cough, or any painful injection site; the baby is healthy.

PE VS: tachycardia (HR 110); mild tachypnea (RR 20); normal BP; fever (38.9°C). PE: breast examination normal; chest exam normal; **uterine tenderness**; lochia staining pad is purulent and foul-smelling; surgical wound clean, dry, and intact.

Labs CBC: **leukocytosis**. UA: trace albumin. **High vaginal swab was stained and cultured**; Gram stain reveals gram-positive cocci and gram-negative bacilli; culture shows **group B streptococci, *Escherichia coli*, and anaerobic peptostreptococci**; blood culture is sterile.

Pathogenesis Puerperal sepsis is caused by normal bacteria in the vaginal flora, which may become pathogenic during the puerperium (due to alteration in normal defenses) or from exogenous pathogens. Diagnosis is clinical with findings of fever (> 100.4°F or 38°C for at least 2 of the first 10 days of the puerperium, excluding the first 24 hours), elevated WBC count, and uterine tenderness.

Epidemiology Risk factors include **early rupture of the membranes, prolonged labor, numerous vaginal examinations, use of internal monitoring devices, and instrumental and operative deliveries such as cesarean section**.

Management Antibiotic treatment includes a combination of an **aminoglycoside** (for gram-negative bacilli), a **third-generation cephalosporin** (for gram-positive and resistant gram-negative coverage), and **metronidazole** (for anaerobic coverage); heparin is administered for septic pelvic thrombophlebitis. In addition to antibiotics, **D&C may be required** to remove retained products of conception.

Complications **Sepsis**, acute renal failure, septic **pelvic thrombophlebitis**, shock and death.

CASE 48

OBSTETRICS

ID/CC A 4-month-old male is brought to a physician with a **bluish rash on his face and trunk**.

HPI The child has had yellowing of the eyes and failure to gain weight. In addition, he has been **behaving as though he were deaf**. There is a history of a **maternal rash** (maculopapular) **during the first trimester**. The mother did not receive prenatal care.

PE Growth retardation; **microcephaly** and bulging anterior fontanelle; **icterus; "blueberry muffin" skin lesions; microphthalmia with cataract** of left eye; discrete **black patchy pigmentation in retina; hepatosplenomegaly**; continuous cardiac "**machinery murmur**."

Labs LFTs: increased direct and indirect serum bilirubin. **Rubella virus isolated** from urine and saliva; **IgM-specific rubella antibody positive**; bilateral **sensorineural deafness**.

Imaging XR, bones: metaphyseal lucent bands and trabecular irregularity extending longitudinally from the epiphysis (**"celery-stalk" appearance**). Echo (with Doppler): **PDA**.

Pathogenesis Rubella virus is an **RNA togavirus** that crosses the placenta. Congenital rubella syndrome has a multiorgan manifestation in which cardiac malformations (PDA, intra-VSD, pulmonary artery stenosis), ocular lesions (cataracts, microphthalmos, chorioretinitis), and CNS abnormalities (mental retardation, microcephaly, deafness) are common. Malformation of bone metaphyses may also be present, with hepatosplenomegaly, thrombocytopenia, thrombocytopenic purpura, interstitial pneumonitis, and myocarditis. **Congenitally affected infants may shed virus for several months and need to be isolated until viral cultures are negative**.

Epidemiology Fetal abnormalities are **most likely to occur if maternal infection is within the first 2 months of gestation**. Immune status testing should be performed for women of childbearing age and for hospital employees who have no history of rubella vaccination. Individuals who are seronegative **should be vaccinated when not pregnant**.

Management No specific antiviral therapy is available; appropriate treatment for specific defects is recommended. Vaccinate immediately postpartum. Contraception should be used for 3 months after vaccination in light of the risk of fetal transmission.

Complications See Pathogenesis.

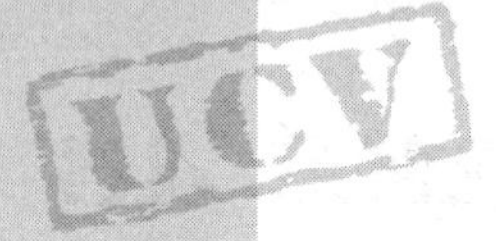

CASE 49

ID/CC A 35-year-old woman complains of **infrequent menstrual bleeding** occurring at > 40-day intervals (OLIGOMENORRHEA) coupled with **cold intolerance, coarse hair**, episodes of sweating with lightheadedness and weakness (due to hypoglycemia), **weight loss** (6 kg in 3 months), and a feeling of constant **fatigue**.

HPI The patient suffered an **abruptio placentae** 7 years ago (average delay for onset of symptoms), with **severe bleeding** followed by **hypovolemic shock**. She had **failure of lactation** and quick breast involution (most common presenting sign) following the pregnancy. She had **persistent amenorrhea** for a year.

PE VS: **hypotension** (BP 100/50); tachycardia (HR 104); no fever. PE: dry skin; **coarse hair**; slow speech; thick tongue; periorbital swelling; **delayed relaxation phase of DTRs**, especially ankle (due to hypothyroidism); **lack of axillary and pubic hair** (due to adrenal insufficiency); vaginal exam reveals atrophic mucosa (due to lack of gonadotropin).

Labs CBC: normocytic, normochromic anemia; lymphocytosis; eosinophilia (due to adrenal insufficiency). **Low prolactin and cortisol; low T_4 and estradiol levels; low ACTH and TSH; low gonadotropins; failure of growth hormone to increase** (to > 7 ng/mL) **after insulin-induced hypoglycemia** (to < 40 mg/dL or to 50% of blood glucose level) (most common laboratory abnormality in hypopituitarism); IV TRH fails to stimulate TSH and prolactin secretion. Lytes: hyponatremia; hyperkalemia (due to decreased aldosterone). ABGs: metabolic acidosis (due to adrenal insufficiency).

Imaging MR, head: the sella turcica fails to show neoplastic or infiltrative involvement.

Pathogenesis Sheehan's syndrome is a result of **ischemia following severe obstetric hemorrhage with necrosis of the anterior pituitary gland**. It is frequently associated with abruptio placentae and coagulopathy. After destruction of the pituitary gland, growth hormone, gonadotropic, thyroid, adrenal, and lactation (prolactin) functions are lost. Symptoms may be delayed for months or years.

Management **Thyroid hormone** (thyroxine), **estrogen**, and **corticosteroid replacement**. Rule out pituitary tumor. Early detection is key.

Complications Infertility, metabolic derangements, and addisonian crisis.

CASE 50

ID/CC A newborn is evaluated for **congenital malformations**.

HPI The mother is a **chronic smoker** but does not abuse alcohol or other drugs; she had no skin rashes or viral prodrome during pregnancy. Routine prenatal tests, including rubella antibody titers, were negative. The baby had a **low birth weight**.

PE Baby appears **small for age; microcephaly** and **cleft lip** present.

Pathogenesis Effects are due to a direct fetoplacental effect of nicotine and its metabolites as well as to reduced fetal oxygenation.

Management Strongly **discourage cigarette smoking**, especially during subsequent pregnancies.

Complications Complications of smoking during pregnancy include increased risk of spontaneous abortion, IUGR, prematurity, **low birth weight, microcephaly**, cleft lip and palate, **placenta previa**, placental abruption, **preeclampsia**, and premature and prolonged rupture of membranes. Maternal cigarette smoking is one of the most common **preventable risk factors for late fetal demise**. There is a long-term relationship between smoking during pregnancy and retarded intellectual development of offspring, sudden infant death syndrome (SIDS), respiratory difficulties, and ADHD.

CASE 51

ID/CC A 29-year-old G1P0 at 37 weeks' gestation presents with severe **headache, visual impairment**, and dull **right upper quadrant abdominal** pain of 4 hours' duration; while in the ambulance, she had a generalized tonic-clonic **seizure**.

HPI She is an otherwise healthy **Hispanic** immigrant of **low socioeconomic status** and is in the ninth month of her **first pregnancy** (primigravida); 2 months ago her family practitioner treated her for **hand and face edema, high blood pressure, and proteinuria** (PREECLAMPSIA). Over the past 3 weeks she has noted **rapid weight gain** (due to edema).

PE VS: **tachycardia** (HR 102); **hypertension** (BP 160/100); no fever. PE: **eyelid and facial edema** (2+); funduscopy reveals **AV nicking**; hyperpigmentation of face (CHLOASMA); chest clear; abdominal exam reveals term uterus; fetal tachycardia (HR 170); right upper quadrant tenderness; no hepatomegaly; **leg edema 3+**; brisk DTRs.

Labs CBC: **increased hematocrit** (hemoconcentration); normal platelets (thrombocytopenia present in HELLP syndrome). **Hyperuricemia**. ABGs: mild acidosis. UA: marked **proteinuria**. LFTs: ALT and AST mildly elevated. Fibrinogen normal (may be decreased in associated abruptio placentae); PT/PTT: normal. Lytes: normal. BUN and creatinine normal (may be increased in associated abruptio placentae).

Imaging CXR: normal (no signs of aspiration pneumonia). CT, head: cerebral edema; no focal lesion.

Pathogenesis Preeclampsia refers to the triad of **hypertension** (increase in systolic blood pressure of > 30 mmHg or 15 mmHg diastolic above baseline level or BP > 140/90), **proteinuria**, and **nondependent edema** (> 5-lb gain/week) from the 20th week of pregnancy to 1 week postpartum. **Eclampsia refers to convulsions in a preeclamptic woman** that cannot be explained by any other etiology; 25% of eclampsia seizures occur antepartum, 50% intrapartum, and 25% postpartum. The etiology of preeclampsia is unknown, but women with hypertension, diabetes, or collagen vascular, autoimmune, or renal disease prior to pregnancy are at increased risk of developing preeclampsia and eclampsia.

Epidemiology Occurs in approximately 1 in 2,000 pregnancies; more frequently seen among younger primigravidae of low socioeconomic groups and among Hispanics and blacks. Mortality is approximately 1%.

Management Prevent and treat convulsions with slow administration of **magnesium sulfate** to prevent concomitant hypotension as a side effect. Magnesium toxicity is monitored by hourly measurement of DTRs, RR and depth, and urine output; toxicity can be counteracted by calcium gluconate.

continued

Diazepam may be used as an adjunctive therapy. If diastolic BP is > 110 mmHg, hydralazine, nifedipine, or labetalol may be used to keep diastolic BP around 90 to 100 mmHg. The definitive treatment of eclampsia is **early delivery** through either induction of labor or cesarean section.

Complications

Fetal complications include premature delivery, growth retardation, periventricular hemorrhage, necrotizing enterocolitis, and abruptio placentae. **Maternal complications** include airway obstruction, postaspiration pneumonia, convulsions, fluid overload, hypoxia, acute renal failure, hepatic capsule rupture, and DIC.

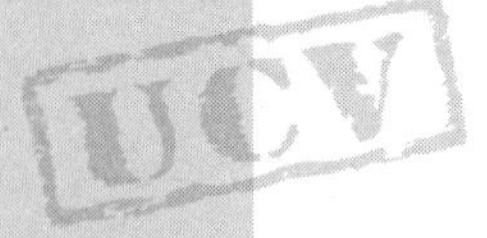

CASE 52

ID/CC A 30-year-old primigravida at 32 weeks' gestation complains of **swelling around the eyes and over her feet**.

HPI She initiated prenatal care at 12 weeks' gestation. **Ultrasound at 18 weeks revealed a twin pregnancy**; subsequent ultrasound at 24 weeks revealed the presence of **hydramnios**. No congenital malformations were found in either fetus.

PE VS: **tachycardia** (HR 110); **hypertension** (BP 140/90); mild tachypnea (RR 20); no fever. PE: **pedal edema; fundal height corresponds to 36 weeks** (more than calculated period of gestation); multiple fetal parts felt; two fetal hearts heard by two different examiners; rates differed by at least 10 beats/minute.

Labs CBC: normal. UA: **proteinuria ++**; 24-hour urine collection contained 900 mg of protein. **Serum uric acid elevated**.

Imaging US, abdomen: gross **polyhydramnios**; the **first twin is vertex, second is breech**; on the basis of measurements of head circumference, abdominal circumference, and biparietal diameter, the second twin **reveals evidence of intrauterine growth retardation**.

Pathogenesis **Monozygotic twins with monochorionic placenta can develop twin-twin** (FETO-FETAL) **transfusion syndrome**. Vascular communication between the twins can result in one fetus with hypervolemia, cardiomegaly, glomerulotubular hypertrophy, ascites, and edema and the other with hypovolemia, growth restriction, and oligohydramnios.

Epidemiology Without assisted fertility, the incidence of twin gestation is about 1 in 80, with 30% monozygotic; the incidence has increased with assisted fertility, both with induction of ovulation with clomiphene and with in vitro fertilization where multiple embryo transfer is undertaken.

Management Concordant twins should be evaluated for growth with US every 4 weeks beginning at 24 weeks. At 36 weeks, patients should be evaluated with non-stress tests and biophysical profiles twice weekly. Discordant twins are tested more often and are delivered at onset of lung maturity or fetal distress.

Complications Complications include **preterm labor, placenta previa, cord prolapse, postpartum hemorrhage, gestational diabetes, polyhydramnios, pre-eclampsia, and anemia**. The fetuses are at an increased risk of congenital malformations, low birth weight, and malpresentation.

ANSWER KEY

1. Bacterial Vaginosis
2. Breast—Intraductal Papilloma
3. Breast Carcinoma
4. Cervical Carcinoma
5. Chancroid
6. Choriocarcinoma
7. Disseminated Gonorrhea
8. Dysfunctional Uterine Bleeding
9. Endometrial Carcinoma
10. Endometriosis
11. Human Papillomavirus (HPV)
12. Hydatidiform Mole
13. Infertility
14. Menopause
15. OCP-Related Cerebrovascular Accident
16. Ovarian Cancer
17. Ovarian Teratoma
18. Pelvic Inflammatory Disease
19. Pelvic Tuberculosis
20. Polycystic Ovary Disease
21. Premenstrual Dysphoric Disorder
22. Primary Amenorrhea—Testicular Feminization
23. Primary Amenorrhea—Turner's Syndrome
24. Rape
25. Reversal of Tubal Ligation
26. Secondary Amenorrhea—Prolactinoma
27. Toxic Shock Syndrome (TSS)
28. Uterine Fibroids
29. Uterine Prolapse with Cystocele
30. Vaginitis—Candidal
31. Vaginitis—*Trichomonas*
32. Vulvar Carcinoma
33. Abortion—Spontaneous
34. Amniotic Fluid Embolism
35. Anemia—Iron Deficiency
36. Anemia of Pregnancy
37. Cholestatic Jaundice of Pregnancy
38. Chorioamnionitis
39. Diabetes in Pregnancy
40. Diagnosis of Pregnancy
41. Ectopic Pregnancy
42. Hyperemesis Gravidarum
43. Placenta Previa
44. Placental Abruption
45. Polyhydramnios
46. Pregnancy with IUD
47. Puerperal Sepsis
48. Rubella—Congenital
49. Sheehan's Syndrome
50. Smoking During Pregnancy
51. Toxemia of Pregnancy—Eclampsia
52. Twin Pregnancy

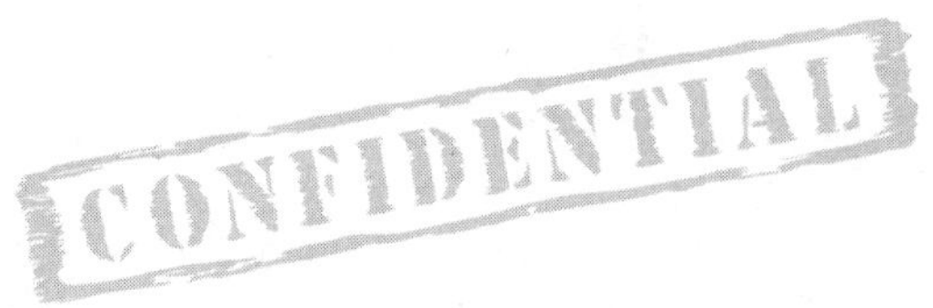

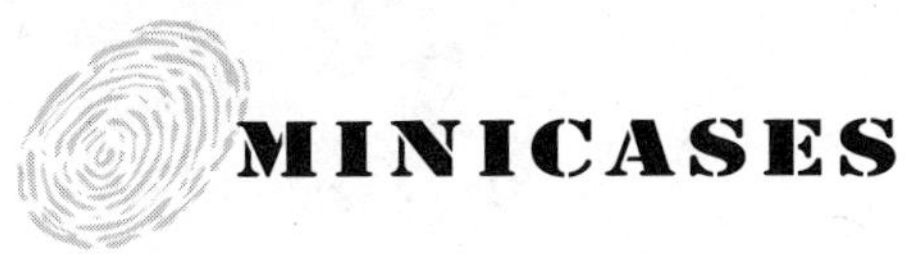

MINICASES

MINICASE 1: Hirsutism—Idiopathic

Male-pattern hair growth in women with normal menses, normal ovaries, and normal adrenal function

- diagnosis of exclusion
- physical exam shows excess facial and body hair
- elevated plasma testosterone and androstenedione levels
- treat with antiandrogens (cimetidine, flutamide) and cosmetic treatment

MINICASE 2: RH Incompatibility

Rh-negative mother produces anti-D antibodies to Rh-positive infant, producing hemolysis and cyanosis in the newborn in the first few hours after birth

- presents with edema, jaundice, and cyanosis in newborn
- positive direct Coombs' test and increased indirect bilirubin
- treat with UV lamp therapy and exchange transfusion

MINICASE 3: Adnexal Torsion

Associated with ovarian tumor or cyst

- presents with abrupt, severe lower abdominal pain and mild fever
- leukocytosis is often seen
- laparoscopy is both diagnostic and therapeutic
- complications include adnexal infarction

MINICASE 4: Breast—Cystosarcoma Phyllodes

A large fibroepithelial tumor of the breast with rapidly growing stroma

- 1 in 4 is malignant
- presents with a palpable breast mass
- treat with wide excision or mastectomy if the size of the tumor precludes lumpectomy

MINICASE 5: Breast—Fibrocystic Disease

Considered a normal breast variant

- patients are usually 30 to 50 years of age
- presents with characteristic micronodular breast texture without discrete lesions
- may have menstrual-related breast pain
- biopsy shows cystic change, adenosis, and fibrosis
- treat for symptomatic relief
- rule out malignancy (by mammography and cyst aspiration of dominant cysts)
- medications used with varying success include progestins, tamoxifen, diuretics, OCPs, and danazol

MINICASE 6: Breast—Paget's Disease

Aggressive breast cancer with overlying skin erythema

- presents with itching, burning, and nipple discharge
- superficial erosion and eczematous scaling may be apparent
- biopsy shows Paget cells invading the dermis
- requires surgical excision

MINICASE 7: Breast Abscess

A localized collection of pus usually associated with lactation

- presents with fever and a tender, erythematous, and fluctuant breast lump that may be draining pus
- leukocytosis, *Staphylococcus aureus* seen on culture of pus
- treat with penicillinase-resistant antibiotics and surgical drainage
- complications include fistula formation

MINICASE 8: Breast Fibroadenoma

The most common benign neoplasm of the female breast, usually seen in young women

- presents with rapid-onset, characteristically round, firm, discrete, movable, nontender nodule in the breast
- US shows solid mass

- biopsy reveals fibrosis
- treat with surgical excision

MINICASE 9: Cervical Polyps

Benign growths

- may be pedunculated or sessile
- present with prolapse of soft, red lesions through the cervix
- may cause postcoital bleeding
- treat by removal
- can use D&C for sessile polyps

MINICASE 10: Cervicitis

Infection of the cervix caused by *Chlamydia, Neisseria gonorrhoeae,* or herpesvirus

- presents with itching or burning with mucopurulent discharge or may be asymptomatic
- pelvic exam reveals red, inflamed cervix and cervical motion tenderness
- cytology reveals atypical epithelial cells and inflammatory cells
- treat with doxycycline and cephalosporin, treat partner as well

MINICASE 11: Dysmenorrhea

Pain associated with menstruation that may be primary or secondary to demonstrable pathology (endometriosis, adenomyosis, fibroids, chronic salpingitis, IUD use, cervical stenosis)

- presents with cramping lower abdominal pain and dyspareunia (usually with secondary dysmenorrhea)
- pelvic exam is unremarkable in primary dysmenorrhea, but in secondary dysmenorrhea it may demonstrate organic pathology (uterine or adnexal tenderness, fixed uterine retroflexion, uterosacral nodularity, a pelvic mass, or an enlarged, irregular uterus)
- labs are normal
- treat primary dysmenorrhea with naproxen or combination OCPs and secondary dysmenorrhea with management of the specific underlying pathology

MINICASE 12: Meigs' Syndrome

A syndrome associated with ovarian fibroma, ascites, and pleural effusions

- presents with dyspnea and pleuritic chest pain
- CXR reveals pleural effusion
- thoracocentesis reveals ovarian fibroma cells
- pelvic US reveals ovarian mass
- treat with therapeutic thoracocentesis, diuresis, treat underlying fibroma with excision

MINICASE 13: Mittelschmerz

Physiologic pelvic pain associated with ovulation

- characteristically presents at midcycle with short-duration, acute, aching abdominal pain
- usually no treatment is required
- NSAIDs, OCPs (to suppress ovulation) may be used in severe cases

MINICASE 14: Ovarian Cyst—Corpus Luteum (Ruptured)

Rupture of corpus luteum cysts

- presents with unilateral abdominal pain and adnexal tenderness
- negative β-hCG
- US may reveal evidence of ruptured cyst
- treat with laparoscopic or open surgery to control bleeding

MINICASE 15: Tubo-Ovarian Abscess

A collection of pus in the fallopian tubes spreading to the ovaries secondary to salpingitis

- commonly caused by *Chlamydia trachomatis* or *Neisseria gonorrhoeae*, but abscess contains mixed aerobic/anaerobic organisms
- presents with fever, abdominal pain, and a palpable adnexal mass on bimanual exam
- leukocytosis and pyuria
- US and CT show the presence of an inflammatory mass in the adnexa

- treatment is doxycycline and cefotetan, with large abscesses requiring surgical excision
- complications include peritonitis and generalized sepsis

MINICASE 16: Vaginitis—Atrophic

Results from estrogen withdrawal (e.g., menopause)

- presents with dyspareunia, white discharge (leukorrhea), pruritus, and punctate vaginal mucosal hemorrhages
- treat with topical estrogen

MINICASE 17: Vulvar Leukoplakia

Disorders of the vulvar epithelium

- causes include vitiligo, malignancies, dystrophies, and inflammatory processes
- presents with genital discoloration and pruritus
- biopsy reveals the underlying cause
- treatment varies with etiology

MINICASE 18: Abortion—Completed

Spontaneous passage of the entire conceptus with closure of the cervix and reduction of the uterus to normal size

- presents with passage of fresh blood, blood clots, and entire conceptus via introitus
- US confirms abortion
- administer RhoGAM in Rh-negative women
- treat by D&C and refer for psychological counseling
- complications include painful cramping and hemorrhage

MINICASE 19: Abortion—Incomplete

Spontaneous passage of part of the conceptus

- presents with passage of fresh blood, blood clots, variable portions of fetal tissue via the introitus, and abdominal cramping

- US confirms lack of fetal heartbeats and rupture of membrane
- treatment is D&C to complete abortion (can wait several days to see if the abortion completes itself spontaneously)
- administer RhoGAM in Rh-negative women
- refer for psychological counseling

MINICASE 20: Abortion—Missed

Retention of dead fetus in utero for several weeks

- presents with failure of uterine expansion on serial examinations or failure to detect fetal heart tones
- US confirms the diagnosis
- treatment is induction of abortion with prostaglandin or with oxytocin (up to 28 weeks)
- complications include dead fetus syndrome, which presents in the second trimester with DIC

MINICASE 21: Acute Fatty Liver of Pregnancy

Unknown etiology

- occurs in the third trimester
- presents with abdominal pain, jaundice, nausea, and vomiting
- elevated PT/PTT, bilirubin, and transaminases
- requires immediate delivery
- complications include hepatic encephalopathy

MINICASE 22: HELLP Syndrome

A variant of eclampsia

- presents with hemolysis, elevated liver enzymes, and low platelets
- definitive treatment is delivery

MINICASE 23: HIV Transmission in Pregnancy

Vertical transmission of HIV most commonly occurring in the third trimester or during birth

- presents with acute retroviral syndrome (e.g., fever, malaise, adenopathy) in the first months of life
- PCR detection of HIV from newborn's blood
- prevention of transmission is the goal of treatment
- giving AZT to the mother during the third trimester or at least during labor markedly diminishes the rate of transmission (from 24% to 8%)

MINICASE 24: Intrahepatic Cholestasis of Pregnancy

Unclear etiology, possibly related to increased estrogen, progesterone

- self-limited and often recurs with pregnancy
- presents with jaundice and pruritus
- bilirubin moderately elevated
- treat with cholestyramine

MINICASE 25: Labor and Delivery

Process by which contractions of a pregnant uterus cause birth, beginning with effacement and dilatation of the cervix and ending with delivery of the placenta

- presents with abdominal enlargement, quickening and lightening, bloody show (expulsion of the mucous plug from the cervix), a sensation of impending defecation, breakage of the amniotic sac, cervical effacement, and crowning of the baby's head
- US may be used to assess fetal position, cardiac activity, and malformations, as well as to estimate fetal weight
- treat by giving oxygen, obtaining IV access, and preparing the field for delivery
- oxytocin may be given to induce uterine contractions
- complications include amniotic fluid embolism, infection, dystocia, malpresentation, umbilical cord complications, and uterine inversion and rupture

MINICASE 26: Postpartum Hemorrhage

Peripartum hemorrhage (blood loss of 500 mL or more within 24 hours of delivery, or any amount of bleeding that is sufficient to produce a hemodynamic compromise) due to uterine atony (the most common cause), retained placenta, or soft tissue injury

- presents with uncontrolled bleeding immediately after delivery, hypotension, and tachycardia, with the uterus boggy and enlarged
- CBC shows anemia, normal coagulation profile
- treat with uterine massage and bimanual uterine compression, oxytocin infusion, and removal of intrauterine clots
- complications include hypovolemic shock and Sheehan's syndrome

QUESTIONS

1. A 20-year-old primigravid comes to you for her first prenatal visit at 12 weeks. She works in a daycare facility and developed a maculopapular rash at 11 weeks' gestation. It disappears after 3 days and she feels fine.

    A. You should reassure her since the symptoms were mild.
    B. Offer termination of the pregnancy.
    C. Obtain her rubella IgG titer.
    D. Obtain a throat culture and treat with penicillin for 10 days.
    E. Obtain a toxoplasmosis IgG titer.

2. At 32 weeks' EGA, a 26-year-old multipara has been hospitalized for 10 days for PROM. She had a previous LTCS because of arrested dilation. For 2 hours she has had light vaginal bleeding and contractions every 15 minutes. Over the past 30 minutes the bleeding has increased slightly, and she experiences lower abdominal pain between contractions. Her temperature is 37.0°C (98.6°F). The uterus is tender and the FHR is 170. Platelet count is 130K, leukocyte count is 14.3K, serum fibrinogen is 225 mg/dL, and the assay for fibrin split products is positive. Which of the following is the most likely diagnosis?

    A. Complete placenta previa
    B. Chorioamnionitis
    C. Abruptio placentae
    D. Uterine scar dehiscence
    E. HELLP syndrome

3. A concerned mother brings in her 16-year-old daughter because she hasn't ever had a menstrual period. On exam, the girl is 5 feet 8 inches tall with mature adult breast development and scant to no pubic nor axillary hair. Vaginal exam is difficult and you are unable to identify a cervix or palpate a uterus. The most likely diagnosis is:

    A. Androgenital syndrome
    B. Imperforate hymen
    C. Turner syndrome
    D. Complete androgen insensitivity syndrome
    E. Rokitansky Kuster Hauser syndrome

4. In evaluating a reproductive age woman who presents with amenorrhea, which of the following conditions will result in a positive (withdrawal) progesterone challenge test?

    A. Pregnancy
    B. Ovarian failure
    C. Pituitary failure
    D. Müllerian agenesis
    E. Polycystic ovary (PCO) syndrome

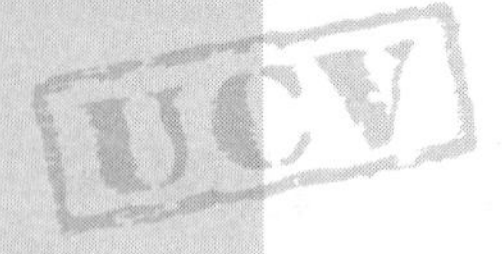

5. A 35-year-old woman presents to your office. She and her 32-year-old husband have been unsuccessful in their attempts to get pregnant for the last 6 years. He has fathered two children in a prior marriage and has a normal semen analysis. Her basal body temperature chart is biphasic. Her past history notes multiple episodes of chlamydia and gonorrhea. A hysterosalpingogram demonstrates blocked fallopian tubes bilaterally, and a laparoscope notes dense and profuse peritubal and pelvic adhesions, along with bilateral clubbed tubes. The most appropriate fertility treatment would be:
   - A. Intrauterine insemination with husband's sperm (IUI)
   - B. Intracytoplasmic sperm injection with husband's sperm (ICSI)
   - C. Gonadotropin induction of ovulation
   - D. *In vitro* fertilization (IVF)
   - E. Gamete intrafallopian transfer (GIFT)

6. A 16-year-old girl presents to your office for gynecologic evaluation. She has never had any vaginal bleeding. She does not recall ever having started her breast development, nor has she had any growth of axillary or pubic hair. Her height is 59 inches. On routine physical exam you see cubitus valgus of the elbows, excess skin of the neck, and a shield-shaped chest with wide-spaced nipples. What is the most appropriate next step in her evaluation?
   - A. Hormone replacement therapy
   - B. Growth hormone therapy
   - C. Estradiol serum level
   - D. Pelvic ultrasonography
   - E. Gonadotropin levels

7. You are asked to see a young woman in the Emergency Department after an alleged sexual assault that occurred today. She is an otherwise healthy 28 years old. A serum pregnancy test is negative. Her menstrual cycle is regular, every 28 days, and her last period was 14 days ago. She is not currently on contraception and desires to minimize her chance of becoming pregnant from this episode. Of the following, the best option is:
   - A. Immediate placement of a copper bearing intrauterine device
   - B. Give Ovral 2 tablets followed by two more tablets 12 hours later.
   - C. Start a daily low dose triphasic birth control pill.
   - D. Start diethylstilbestrol (DES) 50 mg per day for 5 days.
   - E. Immediate dilation and suction curettage

8. A 23-year-old sexually active woman with a prior history of pelvic inflammatory disease presents with sudden onset of pelvic pain. On initial workup and exam, you note the following: Beta HCG titer 5,400 mIU/ml; WBC 4,500 (units); differential: 63 PMNs, 0 Bands, 37 lymphocytes; temperature 37.3°C (99.1°F). An endovaginal ultrasound shows nothing in the uterus, a 2-cm simple left ovarian cyst, and moderate free fluid in the cul-de-sac. The most likely diagnosis is:

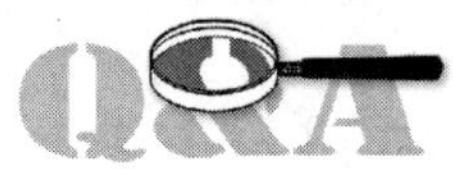

A. Recurrent pelvic inflammatory disease
B. Ectopic pregnancy
C. Ruptured ovarian cyst
D. Endometriosis
E. Irritable bowel syndrome

9. Mixing vaginal discharge with potassium hydroxide (KOH) creates an odor that is helpful in diagnosing:

A. Bacterial vaginosis
B. Trichomoniasis
C. Moniliasis
D. Gonorrhea
E. Chlamydia

10. Three days after her menses started, this 21-year-old woman began having sudden onset of nausea, vomiting, diarrhea, and a flu-like malaise. She does not use tampons, but has had sexual relations in the last several days and uses a cervical cap for contraception. On evaluation, you find her blood pressure to be 75/35 mmHg, pulse of 130 bpm, and an oral temperature of 39.3°C (102.7°F). She has a diffuse macular rash over her entire body. Of the following, which is correct?

A. Blood cultures will be positive for *Staphylococcus aureus.*
B. Blood cultures will be positive for *Neisseria gonorrhoeae.*
C. Most of the clinical signs and symptoms are due to a bacterial endotoxin.
D. Intravenous fluid resuscitation to correct hypotension is the first priority in therapy.
E. Beta lactamase-resistant penicillin antibiotic therapy is the first priority in therapy.

11. A 52-year-old woman presents to your office complaining of vaginal bleeding. Her last bleeding episode was 2 years ago. She is not on hormone replacement therapy. Her hemoglobin is 13.4. A vaginal ultrasound shows her uterus and adnexa to be normal size and an endometrial stripe of 11 mm. The next step in her evaluation should be:

A. Hysterectomy
B. Dilation and curettage
C. Endometrial biopsy
D. Endometrial ablation
E. Intermittent progestin therapy

12. A 19-year-old primigravid at 40 weeks' gestation has been in labor for the last 8 hours. Fetal heart tones have a baseline of 135/min with normal variability, multiple accelerations, and no decelerations. She has been completely dilated for the last hour, and with pushing, has descended from a +1 station

to a +3 station at present. The vertex is direct occiput anterior. Your next course of action is to recommend:

A. Forceps-assisted vaginal delivery
B. Vacuum-assisted vaginal delivery
C. Continue to push
D. Pitocin augmentation
E. Cesarean section

13. A 27-year-old woman presents to your gynecology clinic for an annual exam. She has not had an exam for 3 years, but has never had any problems prior. She presents because she is interested in birth control as she is now in a monogamous sexual relationship. As part of this routine exam you perform a Pap smear, do testing for gonorrhea and *Chlamydia*, and start her on a monophasic oral contraceptive pill. The Pap smear returns with a result of mild dysplasia/low-grade squamous intraephithelial lesion/CIN I. You meet with her 2 weeks later to discuss the ramifications of this finding. You tell her the following in your discussion:

A. With CIN I, the average length of time to the development of cervical cancer is 3–4 years.
B. Seventy percent of CIN I lesions resolve spontaneously.
C. The next step in management is cryotherapy.
D. Cervical dysplasia is highly associated with HPV subtypes 16 and 18.
E. The next step in management is laser therapy.

14. A 46-year-old GO obese woman with chronic hypertension and diabetes presents with infiltrating ductal carcinoma of the breast. She undergoes a wide local excision and axillary lymph-node dissection. Surgery is performed without complications and there is no evidence of metastatic disease on the frozen section. You go to the postoperative area to discuss these findings with her. She is quite bitter about her diagnosis, but glad that she got the disease at age 46 rather than at age 42 like her sister who had bilateral disease requiring mastectomies. She asks you why she got breast cancer. You tell her which of the following was her strongest risk factor:

A. Obesity
B. Nulliparity
C. Hypertension
D. Family history
E. Diabetes

15. A 54-year-old woman presents for an exploratory laparotomy and TAH-BSO for a 7-cm left pelvic mass. Upon entering the abdomen, peritoneal washings are taken. The mass is isolated to the left ovary with no evidence that it is broken beyond the capsule. Upon examination of the uterus, tubes, and contralateral ovary, there is no gross evidence of disease. Upon palpation of the

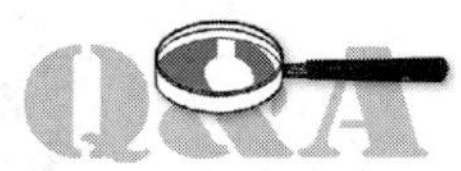

pelvic and aortic lymph nodes, they seem entirely normal. There is no evidence of any lesions on the bowel, omentum, or diaphragm either. Final pathology returns consistent with the above gross findings, but with positive malignant cells in the washings. Given the above tumor and the positive peritoneal washings, what is the stage of this ovarian cancer?

A. Ia
B. Ib
C. Ic
D. IIb
E. IIIc

16. A 32-year-old G2P1 presents at $36^{4}/_{7}$ weeks' GA with a dichorionic/diamniotic twin gestation. Her twin gestation was diagnosed by ultrasound at 8 weeks' GA. An anatomic survey and amniocentesis were performed at 17 weeks' GA, both of which were normal. The fetal karyotypes are 46XY and 46XX. The patient had another ultrasound at 29 weeks' GA, which showed concordant fetal growth with percentile weights of 46 and 57%, respectively. The patient is now presenting with contractions every 2–3 minutes and a cervical exam of 2-cm dilation, 90% effacement, and 0 station. You counsel her that which of the following is commonly accepted in the delivery of twins?

A. Trail of labor for breech presenting twin, cephalic second twin
B. High-dose Pitocin after delivery of the first twin to remove the placenta
C. Immediate delivery of the second twin with forceps, despite the cervix being no longer fully dilated
D. Elective cesarean delivery for a cephalic presenting first twin and cephalic presenting second twin
E. After delivery of the first twin, immediate breech extraction of the second twin

17. A 26-year-old G1P0 presents in active labor at $39^{2}/_{7}$ weeks' GA. She had an uncomplicated antepartum course and has a history of scleroderma. Her disease is currently under control with the use of prednisone. In labor, you begin stress dose steroids. Two hours later, you are called by nursing for a prolonged deceleration. Upon pelvic examination, your note a prolapsed umbilical cord beyond the fetal head. You lift the fetal head off of the cord and the fetal heart rate returns to the 130s. The patient is moved to the operating room for an emergent cesarean delivery as you continue to lift the fetal head off the umbilical cord. In the OR, the obstetric anesthesiologist asks about your preference for anesthesia. You say that:

A. Epidural anesthesia is preferred.
B. Spinal anesthesia is preferred.
C. She needs to be given general anesthesia.
D. You can use local anesthesia with conscious sedation.
E. A pudendal block can be placed.

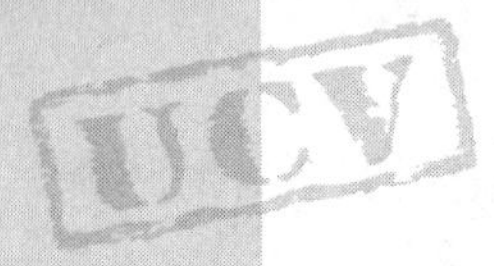

18. A 17-year-old G0 patient presents to the ED with complaints of fever and lower abdominal pain. On physical exam she has a temperature of 101.2°F (38.4°C) and bilateral lower abdominal tenderness. On bimanual exam she has cervical motion tenderness with bilateral adnexal tenderness. There is a slight fullness on her right that is difficult to assess because of her discomfort. She is admitted to the hospital with the diagnosis of PID and started on cefoxitin and doxycycline. After 48 hr of this therapy, she still has fevers to 101.6°F (38.7°C). The next step in management is:

    A. Laparoscopy
    B. Laparotomy
    C. Await final cultures
    D. Pelvic ultrasound
    E. Change antibiotics to ampicillin and gentamicin

19. A 62-year-old woman presents to the ED complaining of two weeks of vaginal spotting. She denies trauma or recent intercourse. Of note, she experienced menopause at age 52, has never been on hormone replacement, and her last Pap smear 3 months ago was normal. On physical exam, she is found to be obese, and pelvic exam reveals an atrophic vagina, a normal-appearing cervix, and a minimal amount of blood in the vaginal vault with no evidence of active bleeding. Her hematocrit is 29 and an endovaginal ultrasound reveals an 8-mm-thick endometrial lining. Which of the following is the next appropriate step in evaluating vaginal bleeding in a postmenopausal woman?

    A. Pap smear to rule out cervical etiologies
    B. Endometrial biopsy to assess the endometrium
    C. Hysteroscopy to search for potential causes of bleeding
    D. Dilation and curettage
    E. Prescribe hormone replacement to stop the bleeding

20. A 17-year-old G3P0-1-1-1 at $32^{5}/_{7}$ weeks' GA present to the ED complaining of moderately painful uterine contractions every 5 min for the past hour. Significant prenatal issues include obesity (prepregnancy weight of 213 lb), history of a prior preterm delivery at 32 weeks' GA, and history of a therapeutic abortion at 11 weeks' GA 3 years ago. Her vital signs are stable, and she is afebrile. On physical exam, she is an obese woman in moderate discomfort but with an otherwise negative exam. Sterile speculum exam and wet mount reveal abundant pseudohyphae, and cervical exam reveals 3 cm dilation and 75% effacement. Which of the following is this patient's biggest risk factor for preterm delivery?

    A. Prior preterm delivery
    B. Prior therapeutic abortion (TAB)
    C. Vaginal candidiasis
    D. Prepregnancy weight
    E. Maternal age

ANSWERS

1. C. If a woman is nonimmune to rubella, then the risk of congenital rubella syndrome is 20% for a primary infection in the first trimester. Cataracts, patent ductus arteriosus, and deafness are the most common findings. In this case, she is coming to you within a few days of having an exanthem; if the patient's rubella IgG shows immunity, then the rash was not due to rubella. If she is rubella IgG negative, then obtain an IgM titer.

   A. Rubella infection in an adult can be a mild viral exanthem. This finding should never be ignored in a pregnant female.
   B. No diagnosis of the condition has been made at this time.
   D. Streptococcal pharyngitis is usually associated with a fever, lymphadenopathy, and pharyngeal symptoms.
   E. Toxoplasmosis is not associated with a maculopapular rash.

2. C. Although this patient has had a prior cesarean section, the possibility of a uterine scar separation is low. With the presence of ruptured membranes, a complete previa is unlikely. Although the uterus is tender, the patient is afebrile. There is literature to suggest that prolonged preterm ROM is associated with an increased risk of abruptio placentae.

   A. Ruptured membranes with a complete previa is very unlikely.
   B. Chorioamnionitis can be a complication of prolonged preterm rupture of membranes. It can be associated with contractions and uterine pain, but is usually not associated with vaginal bleeding.
   D. Uterine scar separation can occur with a prior cesarean, but usually occurs in active labor. This patient is showing signs of early uterine activity at 32 weeks' gestation, making this diagnosis unlikely.
   E. HELLP syndrome is hemolysis, elevated liver enzymes, and low platelets.

3. D. Complete androgen insensitivity syndrome is due to a congenital lack of androgen receptors. The patient never develops the müllerian system since the gonad produces anti-müllerian hormone (AMH or MIF) from the Sertoli cells during organogenesis. Although the patient has a male level of testosterone and male levels of estrogen, since the androgens are not recognized, the breasts develop due to the presence of estrogens. Without androgens, these patients often have sparse to no sexual hair. As the gonad is an XY gonad, it must be removed to prevent the risk of malignant transformation; this is rare prior to puberty, so it can be removed after normal pubertal development has occurred (most common malignancy is a gonadoblastoma).

   A. One would see the effects of excess androgen: hair growth, virilization, etc.
   B. The vagina would be behind the imperforate hymen and not visible. If menses has begun, then there would be a bluish bulging mass (vagina full of old menstrual blood).
   C. A uterus is present in Turner syndrome.

E. Although a uterus is absent in this syndrome, sexual hair should be present since there is no defect in either androgen production or in androgen receptors.

4. **E. In pregnancy, progesterone is produced by the corpus luteum followed by the placenta. Exogenous progesterone will not lead to withdrawal bleeding. In ovarian failure as well as pituitary failure, no estrogen stimulation of the endometrium exists, and progesterone cannot cause withdrawal bleeding. With müllerian agenesis, there is no endometrium. Polycystic ovarian syndrome has an abundance of circulating estrogen, so the endometrium will proliferate.**

A. Progesterone withdrawal will not occur since the corpus luteum is producing progesterone. The placenta will take over, starting at 7 weeks, and will be the sole producer of progesterone by 12 weeks.
B. No estrogen will be produced; no proliferation of the endometrium will occur.
C. Without gonadotropin stimulation, there will not be enough estrogen to stimulate the endometrial lining.
D. There is no uterus, thus no bleeding.

5. **D. With extensive tubal disease on both the HSG and laparoscopy, operative assistance will be needed in order for an egg to reach the uterine cavity. Due to the tubal disease, GIFT is not possible. ICSI is the treatment of choice for azoospermia and severe oligospermia. The patient is ovulatory based on her basal body temperature chart, so ovulation induction alone is not necessary. IVF with transcervical transfer of the embryo is the optimal treatment for this couple. With blastocyst transfer, the current success rates are above 50%.**

A. The two tests of tubal function both demonstrate that it is highly unlikely for the egg to successfully transport down the tube. Thus, IUI will be of no benefit, since the sperm and egg will not meet.
B. ICSI is used for oligospermic and even some azoospermic males to achieve fertilization.
C. Again, ovulation induction alone will not be successful if the tubes are blocked bilaterally.
E. This technique can only be used if there is tubal patency. The egg and sperm mixture is placed in the distal fallopian tube via laparoscopy. The tubes here are blocked.

6. **E. This picture is a classic example of a phenotypic Turner syndrome female. Ninety-nine percent of all monosomy X fetuses will spontaneously abort. Congenital lymphedema in utero leads to the development of a cystic hygroma along with many of the other visible external manifestations. About 60% of Turner patients have total loss of one X chromosome; the remainder have either a structural abnormality in one of the X**

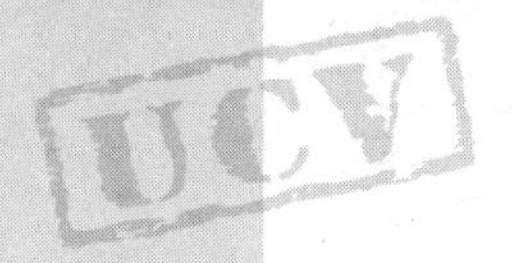

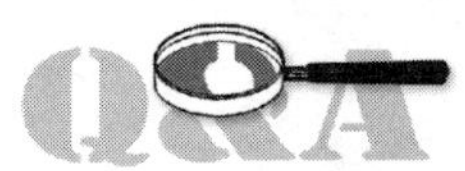

chromosomes or mosaicism with an abnormal X. Other phenotypic findings include a high arched palate, renal abnormalities (horseshoe kidney, partial or complete duplication, etc.), and a low posterior hairline. One-third of these women will have cardiovascular abnormalities (coarctation of the aorta, bicuspid aortic valve, etc.). Autoimmune disorders such as Hashimoto's thyroiditis and Addison's disease are common. The general recommendations are that gonadotropin levels are the first test indicated when the clinical picture of a classic Turner syndrome patient presents. A karyotype will confirm the diagnosis and help determine further recommendations should any Y chromosomal elements exist.

A. This patient will require hormone replacement therapy as she has no ovaries. It is not, however, the next step in the evaluation.
B. Growth hormone therapy in childhood has been suggested to allow these patients to approach near normal height in adulthood. It is controversial at present.
C. As no secondary sexual characteristics due to estrogen have appeared, an estradiol level will not be required.
D. Pelvic ultrasound may demonstrate tissue in the region of the adnexa. The streak gonads measure about 0.5 by 2.0 cm.

7. **B. Currently, postcoital birth control can be done either with an IUD or with hormonal therapy. With OCPs, you need to give two doses, each of at least 100 μg of ethinyl estradiol (2 Ovral). Less than 2% of women will become pregnant with this dose (prevents 75% of expected pregnancies), and it can be given up to 72 hours after coitus. DES has a slightly higher success rate, but due to the significant side effect rate, compliance with this regimen is much less, making it less effective. An IUD is an option if there is no risk for sexually transmitted diseases, so it is not indicated after a sexual assault. Some countries also use two doses of 0.75 mg levonorgestrel, which has a similar success rate to the Ovral regimen. Note that the clinical pregnancy rate of unprotected midcycle coitus is about 7%.**

A. IUDs can be used for emergency postcoital contraception, but are not indicated when the risk for a sexually transmitted disease is present.
C. A minimum of 100 μg of ethinyl estradiol in two divided doses needs to be given.
D. Significant side effects (nausea) make compliance with this regimen much less, making it less effective.
E. At this point, the fertilized ovum is still within the fallopian tube.

8. **B. With her prior history of PID, her chances of tubal damage are significantly elevated. Since she is pregnant with an HCG titer over 2,000 mIU/mL, an intrauterine gestation sac should have been seen on the endovaginal ultrasound. With the moderate amount of free fluid in the**

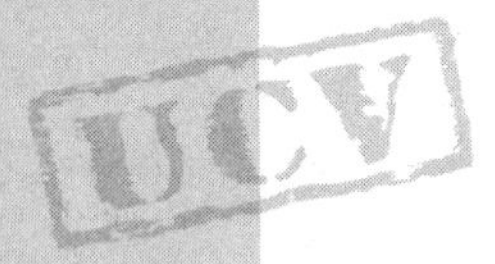

cul-de-sac, along with the pelvic pain and normal white count and temperature, the index of suspicion for an ectopic pregnancy must be high.

A. The white count is normal and her temperature is normal as well. With a positive HCG titer, an ectopic pregnancy should be the first suspicion.
C. This can cause free fluid in the cul-de-sac as well as pelvic pain. With her history of PID in the past, the presence of tubal damage is high, so one should be much more suspicious of an ectopic pregnancy. At an HCG titer of 5,400, an IUP should have been seen.
D. Although a source of pelvic pain, with the HCG titer, absence of an IUP on ultrasound, and free fluid in the cul-de-sac, ectopic pregnancy should be the primary diagnosis.
E. Can be a source of pelvic pain. See answer to D.

9. **A. Bacterial vaginosis is due to an overgrowth of anaerobic bacteria, replacing the normal peroxide-producing *Lactobacillus* species. The discharge is described as thin and gray white in color. It is mildly adherent to the vaginal walls on speculum exam. In the presence of basic environment (semen, KOH), the aromatic amines are released, giving rise to the characteristic fishy odor.**

B. In order to create an odor with a strong base, there must be aromatic amines present. These are created by certain anaerobic bacteria.
C. See answer to B.
D. See answer to B.
E. See answer to B.

10. **D. This is the classic picture for toxic shock syndrome. Although it is more commonly associated with tampon usage, it can occur after use of a contraceptive sponge, diaphragm, or cervical cap. It can also occur postoperatively in a patient with gauze packing. Cultures are usually negative, though *Staphylococcus aureus* is the most common pathogen. An exotoxin is the causative agent for the systemic effects. Correction of circulatory compromise is the most important initial therapy in treating this condition. If a source exists for the bacteria, it must be removed as well (i.e., tampon, etc.).**

A. In most cases of toxic shock syndrome, the causative agent will not be found in the bloodstream.
B. This is not the typical presentation of disseminated gonococcemia.
C. The causative agent for the systemic effects is an exotoxin produced by the bacteria.
E. Correction of circulatory compromise and removal of the bacterial source are the most important initial therapies.

11. **C. In any woman over the age of 35, with abnormal uterine bleeding, the diagnosis of an endometrial malignancy must be entertained. With a**

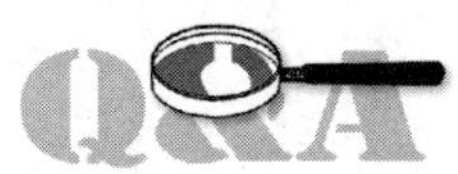

postmenopausal woman having an endometrial stripe over 4 mm, cancer needs to be ruled out and tissue should be obtained. The simplest test is to proceed with an endometrial biopsy.

A. This therapy would be indicated as therapy for adenocarcinoma of the endometrium or for atypical endometrial hyperplasia. A diagnostic sampling of the endometrium is the first necessary test.
B. Although this test would lead to a diagnosis, an endometrial biopsy can be done more easily in the office with minimal discomfort.
D. This modality is used for the reproductive age female with severe symptomatic uterine bleeding in the absence of endometrial pathology.
E. A diagnosis of the endometrium must be made before hormonal therapy can be started in this case.

12. **C. This patient is progressing in normal fashion. She is allowed up to 2 hours in the second stage and even longer if the heart tones are reassuring. There is no need to intervene, and one would anticipate that the patient will be having a normal spontaneous vaginal delivery within the next hour.**

A. The patient has made adequate descent in the last hour. She can push for at least another hour and maybe more if the fetal condition remains reassuring. No indication for instrumental vaginal delivery is present.
B. The patient has made adequate descent in the last hour. She can push for at least another hour and maybe more if the fetal condition remains reassuring. No indication for instrumental vaginal delivery is present.
D. The patient has made adequate descent in the last hour. She can push for at least another hour and maybe more if the fetal condition remains reassuring. Since progress has been made, there is no need to augment the labor with Pitocin.
E. The patient has made adequate descent in the last hour. She can push for at least another hour and maybe more if the fetal condition remains reassuring. No indication for cesarean delivery is present.

13. **D. There is a high association between cervical dysplasia, cervical cancer, and human papillomavirus (HPV). In particular, the subtypes that put one at risk include 16, 18, and 31, whereas subtypes 6 and 11 predispose to condyloma formation.**

A. The average length of time to the development of cervical cancer with CIN I is 7 years, whereas CIN II can develop into carcinoma in 3–4 years. However, there are lesions that progress much faster. Thus, more patients are managed aggressively.
B. Thirty percent of CIN I lesions resolve spontaneously.

C & E. The next step in the management of a CIN I lesion would be scheduled colposcopy and directed biopsy. Colposcopy allows a better view of the cervix and uses acetic acid to bring out the possible lesions by turning them white. Once a formal diagnosis is made, CIN I lesions are usually followed every 3–4 months with colposcopy until the lesion either regresses or progresses. If a diagnosis is made at that time, cryotherapy or laser can be used. However, an excisional procedure that can demonstrate clear margins is often the procedure of choice with either the large loop excision of the transformation zone (LLETZ or LEEP) or a cold-knife-cone biopsy.

14. **D. A first-degree relative with bilateral, premenopausal disease carries an 8-fold increase in breast cancer risk. This family history is the strongest risk factor in any patient, and management usually entails annual mammograms starting 10 years prior to when the relative was diagnosed with the disease.**

A. Obesity carries a relative risk of 2.
B. Nulliparity is associated with a 3-fold risk of disease when compared to parous patients.
C. Hypertension appears associated with breast cancer, with an odds ratio between 1.2 and 1.5.
E. Diabetes, similar to hypertension, is weakly associated with breast cancer.

15. **C. Ovarian cancer stage I is as follows: Ia is confined to one ovary, Ib is both ovaries, Ic is either a or b with rupture of the ovary, disease outside the capsule, or positive peritoneal washings.**

A & B. See C above.
D & E. See below:

<u>Staging of Ovarian Carcinoma</u>

Stage II—Disease extends to the pelvis
a—Malignant cells in the uterus or fallopian tubes
b—Malignant cells elsewhere in the pelvis
c—a or b plus positive washings or disease beyond the capsule

Stage III—Disease extends to the abdomen
a—Only microscopic disease
b—Metastases < 2 cm in size
c—Metastases > 2 cm in size or any positive pelvic or para-aortic nodes

Stage IV—Distant metastases include positive pleural effusion and disease in the liver parenchyma.

16. **E. Twin pregnancies can be dizygotic (two initial zygotes) or monozygotic (one initial zygote that splits into two at some point). Dizygotic twins will always be dichorionic and diamnionic—two placentas and two amniotic cavities. Monozygotic twins can be di/di, mono/di, mono/mono, or conjoint**

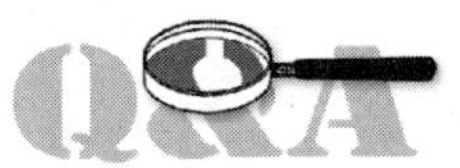

(known by laypersons as Siamese), depending on when the zygote splits. At delivery, twin pregnancies can present in a variety of ways. Each fetus can be cephalic, breech, or transverse, creating nine possible presentations. If the presenting fetus is cephalic and the twins are concordant, a trial of labor with cephalic delivery or breech extraction of the second twin is reasonable.

A. Vaginal delivery of a breech presenting twin followed by a cephalic twin is usually not allowed. In addition to the usual risks of delivering the presenting twin breech, there is a risk of interlocking twins, where the second twin's head comes through the pelvis before the first twin's head.
B. After delivery of the first twin, the uterus rapidly decreases in size, which increases the risk for abruption of the second twin's placenta. Augmentation with high-dose Pitocin is likely to increase the risk of abruption and tetanic contractions. Classically, the occurrence of an undiagnosed twin is the reason Pitocin is not given until after delivery of the placenta.
C. Forceps should never be applied when the cervix is not fully dilated.
D. If both twins are cephalic presenting, there is no indication for cesarean delivery.

17. **B. In the setting of an emergent cesarean delivery, it is reasonable to utilize spinal anesthesia as long as it can be administered quickly (< 5 min) and there is no abruption, uterine rupture, or ongoing cause of severe hypoxia. In this case, given the reassuring fetal heart rate, spinal anesthesia is preferred as the head is lifted off of the cord.**

A. Epidural anesthesia takes longer to achieve a surgical level, and is less often successful than spinal anesthesia. Epidural anesthesia is excellent for labor because continuous administration and titration for less neuromuscular block are possible.
C. In a true emergent cesarean delivery, if the anesthesiologist does not normally place many spinals, general anesthesia is commonly used. This patient may not be a good candidate for intubation, given her history of scleroderma. Hopefully, the patient and her airway were evaluated by anesthesia at admission.
D. Occasionally, if anesthesia is unavailable, a cesarean section will be performed under local anesthesia with conscious sedation. This is certainly not an optimal way to perform surgery, and given the presence of an obstetric anesthesiologist in this case, is unnecessary.
E. Pudendal anesthesia may be administered by an obstetrician prior to performing an operative vaginal delivery with vacuum or forceps.

18. **D. With presumed pelvic inflammatory disease (PID) and no resolution of symptoms or signs after 48 hr of appropriate treatment, the patient is at risk for a tubo-ovarian abscess (TOA). This is best diagnosed by pelvic**

ultrasound. Furthermore, given her symptoms, pelvic ultrasound should probably have been performed on admission to rule out TOA.

A. Laparoscopy is used in some facilities to diagnose PID, but would be of little use at this point in the patient.
B. If the patient has a TOA that does not respond to more aggressive antibiotics, she may require surgical treatment. Because she is a young woman, and surgical management often involves salpingo-oophorectomy, conservative management with antibiotics is usually first-line therapy.
C. Cultures from the cervix can be useful to fine-tune antibiotic treatment. In this patient who is not responding to medical therapy, broadening treatment is likely to be more effective than waiting for culture results.
E. While broadening coverage may be necessary, ampicillin and gentamicin would need to be given with clindamycin for coverage of chlamydia and anaerobic organisms.

19. **B. Approximately 20% of vaginal bleeding in postmenopausal women is due to cancer. In particular, endometrial cancer is the most common gynecologic malignancy in the United States, causing 50–60% of postmenopausal bleeding in women > 80 years. Endometrial biopsy is the gold standard for diagnosing endometrial cancer because of the ease with which it can be performed. However, if this patient were experiencing heavy, ongoing bleeding, a D&C would be more appropriate as it would stop the bleeding and obtain a specimen for pathology.**

A. Cervical etiologies are unlikely in a woman with a recently normal Pap smear and no visible lesion or history of trauma. It is still necessary to rule out cervical cancer as an etiology for bleeding, but the incidence of endometrial cancer is higher and should therefore be investigated first.
C. Although hysteroscopy would be useful in identifying potential causes for bleeding, such as endometrial polyps and myomas, malignant etiologies should be addressed first. Given the thickened endometrium (> 5 mm in postmenopausal women) found on ultrasound, the endometrium should be assessed prior to proceeding with hysteroscopy.
D. See answer B.
E. Given the high likelihood of malignancy, attempting to manage the bleeding medically without first evaluating potential etiologies is inappropriate.

20. **A. Although numerous risk factors exist for preterm delivery, the biggest risk factor is history of a prior preterm delivery. Other risk factors for preterm labor include multiple gestations, polyhydramnios, African**

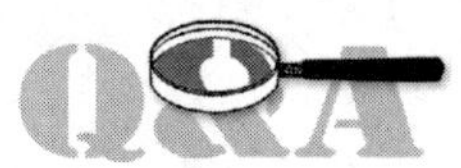

American race, bacterial vaginosis, uterine anomalies, preterm rupture of the membranes, preeclampsia, and some maternal medical conditions.

B. While it has been theorized that multiple TABs increase the risk of incompetent cervix, there have been no studies to date that correlate history of one prior TAB with preterm delivery.

C. Bacterial vaginosis has been associated with preterm labor, but no such association exists with vaginal candidiasis.

D. A prepregnancy weight of < 50 kg is a risk factor for preterm delivery, but no such association exists with obesity.

E. While it is true that maternal age < 20 is associated with preterm delivery, this is not the patient's biggest risk factor.